IT'S A TANGO, NOT A WAR

Dancing with Type 1 Diabetes

D1603352

ISBN 9798985236705 (Paperback edition)
ISBN 9798985236712 (Ebook edition)
Library of Congress Control Number: 2022904186

All examples are real. Some names have been changed. Medical and psychological information was reviewed by professionals.

Cover by Robin Locke Monda
Book design by Asya Blue Design

Printed in the United States of America
First Printing April 2022
Agua Fria Publishing
PO Box 8513
Santa Fe, New Mexico 87504

Visit www.KarenMeadowsDiabetes.com

IT'S A TANGO, NOT A WAR

Dancing with Type 1 Diabetes

KAREN MEADOWS

CONTENTS

Resources at KarenMeadowsDiabetes.com

Acknowledgments

With love to my mother and father. I wish I had better understood all you gave me and thanked you while you were still alive.

I am grateful to all who helped me create and publish this book. Special thanks to my writing coach Jennifer Louden, my 2020 and 2021 Mastermind Writers Groups, my sisters Linda Gross and Nancy Ashworth, Kayleen Chavarillo, Marjorie Cypress, Karen Halderson, Kellie Kirksey, Mindy Meiering, Marge Morris, Abra Patkotak, Bill Polonsky, Annette Tixier, Perdita Wexler, Anthony Willert, and to all my friends and clients.

Disclaimer

The purpose of this book is to help people with type 1 diabetes and those who support them better understand the complexity of this condition. Further, this book is meant to encourage readers to know themselves more deeply and make healthy choices.

Readers are encouraged to work closely with their own medical care teams and to discover what works best for their individualized health plans. The information provided is meant to offer perspective.

The author's expertise comes from her personal experience as a person with type 1 diabetes and a Certified Diabetes Care & Education Specialist. She is not a therapist or a medical professional. The medical information in this book comes from reputable sources that readers can also access online, and was reviewed by medical and psychological professionals. The stories are her own and those of people she knows. The author takes no responsibility for adverse effects resulting from the information found in this book.

Introduction

Welcome.

Are you a human being looking for ways to live well with type 1 diabetes? Do you love someone with type 1 diabetes? Are you a boss, a medical professional, a coach or a curious coworker who wants to understand type 1 diabetes?

These chapters cover crucial topics that have affected me in my 60 years living with type 1. Incorporating medical facts, I describe times when I met or my clients met a health drama, how we responded and what we learned. My hope is that you see yourself in my stories, and love yourself even more for all that you do to stay healthy.

Everything in this book about loving yourself and considering diabetes your ally is true. But I had to go through a final test to believe myself before finishing. I wrote these chapters as the Covid-19 epidemic isolated me. I felt strong and sure after years of thinking about this project. Writing my chapters unfolded without trauma. My book coach and writing circle supported me beautifully. Then it seemed I had no more to write. Advisors said, "You are done now.

Just say 'done' and publish it." I knew I wasn't done but I didn't know why. I felt untethered, unsure.

I began writing this introduction, but I still didn't feel done. Covid was receding in the United States. I had both vaccines. I was pleased to return to counseling patients in my health center, but uncomfortable venturing out into the world again. Then my sister began falling and was moved from her assisted living apartment into a clinical setting. Because she lives far away, I communicated by phone for hours a day with a long line of people helping her. She refused my calls.

My own health took a turn. I read results of my blood and urine tests before meeting with my endocrinologist, and thought they indicated kidney damage. Already feeling lost, I retreated into fear and sorrow and anger.

To shift the tide of bad feelings and physical loss I began using techniques I had learned over the years but put aside. I tapped acupuncture points using a procedure called EFT (Emotional Freedom Technique). Statements begin with *Even though...* and you fill in what you're going through. You end each statement with *...I deeply and completely love and accept myself.* You work from negative thoughts to positive, tapping all the way.

And I used energy medicine educator Donna Eden's daily physical routine for grounding, protecting and healing myself. But still in turmoil I emailed a friend and therapist for help. We agreed to speak at 3 p.m. I told her my sister was angry with me for moving her and getting rid of her possessions. That had catapulted me back into childhood defenses and I was trying desperately to please everyone involved. Meanwhile I felt guilty and ineffective.

Even more worrisome was the state of my kidneys. I leapt into images of a terrible future. Unwilling to endure dialysis, and too old to qualify for a transplant, what would I do if my kidneys failed me? Wicked diabetes was no partner of mine. And finishing my book inviting readers to call type 1 their ally seemed impossible.

Annette listened intently, not interrupting, and then asked, "Do you believe what you've written in this book?"

Damn, that hit home. I *did* believe what I'd written. But fear still tapped at the windows.

"This is all about your destiny, your life purpose, about faith, hope and trust," Annette continued.

"You have lived fully with your diabetes, even *because of* your diabetes. Sometimes it is terrifying but you have stepped into it anyway. You are one of the bravest people I know. All your experience is evidence that you *have* a partnership with your diabetes. Your sister is reminding you who you are. Your kidneys are warning you—before it is too late—that something needs to change. These events are gifts."

I listened and cried.

"Stay in the present," she said. "Listen to your body. It doesn't lie."

The present felt like a terrible place to be. I didn't want to be present with loss and unanticipated change and potential disability—for my sister or myself. And of course I didn't want to step into my body. I didn't want to know what my kidneys had to say to me. I have long assumed that type 1s rightfully leave our bodies just to avoid the stabs of blood sugar lancets and insulin needles.

But as Annette's words poured over me I began to settle both mind and body. I breathed consciously from above my head to below my feet with her and connected more firmly with the earth and myself on it. I renewed my belief that life, especially with type 1 diabetes, is an ongoing process, and I will find my own way.

I am an ordinary person who has lived a very long time with type 1 diabetes. I am a soul experiencing life on earth. My life path has revealed ongoing discovery and evolution. Although there are times I would like to *stop* evolving, that isn't life. I know I must be brave. And you must be brave. Life with type 1 diabetes is hard. We need to stand firm and build strength to meet all that comes our way. We always have choices, and how we manage our diabetes is in our own hands and therefore very personal.

I provide no steps for you to follow. This is not a self-help book. It is a self-awareness book. I invite people with type 1 diabetes to know and celebrate themselves as they are, and to build and enjoy an individualized life and health plan.

Maybe you aren't there yet. Or maybe, like me, you occasionally get lost. You might feel like Charlie Brown's poor little Christmas tree. Look closer. In the movie *Charlie Brown's Christmas* although it was a scrawny specimen, he picked the only real tree in a lot full of perfect metal ones. His friends shamed Charlie Brown and made fun of his tree, but Linus said, "Maybe it just needs a little love." Finally, Charlie's circle of friends surrounded and decorated the little tree, which lit up and became truly beautiful.

When you wonder about yourself and your life with type 1 diabetes (T1D), remember that being human is difficult, and having T1D is especially difficult. But you are real and any steps you take to light up and beautify yourself illuminate the world around you.

You are meant to discover your own path. And you learn from making mistakes along the way. I like to consider this adventure a dance, a precise but ever-changing dance, perhaps a tango.

People with T1D are often categorized as victims *suffering* from an incurable disease! That description does not serve me. I am a capable human with an exacting condition that might actually add value to my life. In partnership with my diabetes, I create the healthy life I want to live.

We are told to fight, but fighting diabetes means fighting ourselves. What about dancing with your complicated, difficult but valuable partner? With diabetes as your ally, you can be stronger and more likely to succeed at whatever you decide to make of yourself.

Here's a simple step you might try right now. Remember a saying, a prayer, an affirmation or mantra that uplifts you, and apply it to your relationship with diabetes. Meditation teacher Jack Kornfield says repeating a mantra affects the very cells of our bodies. One mantra he repeats is, "May I hold all the joys and sorrows of my life with loving kindness."

Experiment. Say to yourself, "May I hold all the joys and sorrows of living with type 1 diabetes with loving kindness." Isn't it tantalizing to even consider the *joys* of living with T1D? Might your life feel more blessed if you treated type 1 diabetes with loving kindness? That is my commitment when I am in the dark. I remembered that commitment when I spoke with Annette.

The greatest, and possibly the only freedom we have, is in our own minds. Let your mind appreciate having diabetes and you may be freer than you could have imagined.

"Diabetes, like COVID-19, is a wicked problem," wrote David Kerr and Namino Glantz in *Lancet*, October 2020. Their article *for doctors* opens with:

> Diabetes has long been mistaken as a tame problem. Following a recipe, playing chess, and doing open-heart surgery are tame problems…. Diabetes, like COVID-19, is a wicked problem…. Wicked problems are impossible to solve because of contradictory and changing requirements, the absence of equality, and ever-evolving social complexities.

Without even designating type 1 diabetes, which I consider much more threatening and misunderstood than type 2, Kerr and Glantz state unequivocally that our condition is wilder than open-heart surgery. I have, and you or someone you know or love has, a wicked unsolvable physical/mental/social condition called type 1 diabetes. How's that for a definition?

You may already know how to live well with the wicked problem called type 1 diabetes. Or not. Either way, as you read this book, one thought, one story, one kernel might burrow into your creative mind and grow into ways to admire and more lovingly care for yourself. Most important to me—you might consider type 1 diabetes an asset to your life on earth. T1D may be the demanding teacher that becomes your best mentor.

Check your blood sugar, put on your dancing shoes and begin to master the tango with T1D. Then settle in and read this book.

With great love, Karen

Notes: The medical world is being wonderfully careful to call us persons with diabetes rather than diabetics. That's a lot of words to repeat over and over again so writers often use the term PWDs. I would have to specify T1PWD or T2PWD. That's awkward and I don't mind being called a T1D or a type 1, so I have used T1D and T2D and type 1 or 2 throughout this book to describe those like me who have a particular condition named diabetes.

Also, one of my medical provider readers advised me to cite more recent journal articles. Although diabetes research is evolving rapidly, when searching for specific information—for example, the presence of complications—I found some valuable information in older sources.

PART 1

MY STORY

CHAPTER 1

In the Beginning

Fall, 1959. There was cholera in the Philippine Islands. My favorite teacher Mr. Baker took our high school geography class to Manila to tour historic sites of the capital. Because of cholera we could not trust the city water, so we drank Pepsi, cold at first but warming as the sultry day moved on. Our U.S. Air Force school bus had no air conditioning. My thirst was unquenchable and the sodas tasted salty and heavy to me. In a plaza under a statue of Filipino national hero José Rizal we ate the lunches our mothers had packed. Later, we were guests at a girls' school where they performed for us, and I watched in agony, needing to pee.

The Philippines is a cluster of tropical islands in Southeast Asia, founded on active volcanoes and ranging from sea level rain forest to mountains higher than 9,000 feet. My father was a U.S. Air Force officer stationed at Clark Air Base. When my family joined him, we lived at first in the summer capital, Baguio, 112 miles from Clark in the mountains.

My parents rented a villa owned by rich Filipinos whose second home, when not rented, provided them with relief from Manila's steaming summer. As Americans, we were thought to be rich too. Our landlady, Mrs. Bautista, visited my mother once and pulled a handkerchief out of her purse. She spilled diamonds onto the coffee table and asked my mother if her friends might like to buy them. Knowing none of her friends could afford diamonds, mother insulted her by laughing.

Baguio was a haven for us, beautiful, cool and hospitable. A short drive away we could look out to the South China Sea. In the city, hill women strolled with baskets of fruit on their heads calling out, "Bananas ma'am?"

Next door lived two boys whose father worked for Voice of America. The boys shared a jeepney ride with me and my sisters every weekday morning. Jouncing to school we hung onto the sides and swayed with the jeepney's bright plastic flowers and bells. Our Catholic school was run by Belgian nuns who were thrilled with us because we asked questions and spoke good English.

With our rented house came a maid, and a houseboy named Toby who polished the patio tiles by skating back and forth on half a coconut shell. On the steep hill above us was a monastery and at dusk a procession of monks wound down the hill chanting their prayers.

Those were blessed months. I flourished in the altitude and the mountains. Filipinos embraced Americans, almost idolizing us— wanting to speak English and learn how we lived. I met a squad of Philippine Military Academy cadets and began receiving, at age 13, ardent love letters. But diabetes was working on me.

After a year in Baguio, our lives changed dramatically. My family moved into military housing at Clark Air Force Base on the plains of central Luzon.

Earthquakes shook us. Typhoons and annual monsoons alternated with drought. We were mostly protected on base, but millions of Filipinos lived in shacks and were regularly swept away. With other Americans I was once flown home on a military plane from visiting a Filipina friend in Manila. Floods had washed out the roads and further threatened the capital city.

As a high school sophomore, I was a cheerleader for Clark's football team, Razor's Orphans (named after the base commander and his men who were far from home and family). In my white sharkskin uniform with red 'O' on my chest I remember chanting, "Rah Rah Ree, kick him in the knee. Rah Rah Rass, kick him in the other knee." I was barely able to keep up. My 5'2" frame had dwindled to 87 pounds and I was exhausted. Type 1 diabetes had arrived but we didn't recognize it.

My parents were distracted. My father flew the general and his aides around Asia and the Middle East. The Vietnam War was building.

Clark Air Base covered 244 square miles, sections quite desolate. When my father had a trip planned, my mother drove him to the flight line in our red VW bug, with a loaded pistol on her lap. Their route wound through an unsecured wooded area where we were told the Hukballahop—*communist insurgents*—might attack. In the housing area, Igorot tribesmen perched in trees every night, protecting our homes with poison blow darts. At school we practiced the *hide under the desk* routine to respond to imagined attack.

The Air Force warriors, all men then, were regularly called out on maneuvers. Wives and children were left behind, told to stay inside. Fear was a constant.

I grew weaker. Mother took me to the base clinic and the doctor who reviewed my symptoms recommended vitamins. He wrote in my chart, "nervous mother." I tried to maintain my activities, but, finally, one Sunday morning I lay in bed, too depleted to go to church.

Attendance at Sunday mass was a strong family ritual. When I couldn't even lift myself out of bed, Dad picked me up and took me to see the flight surgeon—the pilots' doctor. I curled up in a big leather chair, falling into a coma. That doctor didn't even examine me. He heard my father's description, looked at me and told my parents, "Go and get her things. I'm putting her in the hospital. She has diabetes."

Fort Stotsenburg Hospital, where I was admitted, had served wounded soldiers from World War II and been occupied by both the U.S. and Japanese military. After my time in the Philippines, Fort Stotsenburg sheltered injured and dying Vietnam War soldiers. The hospital was profiled in 2019 by the TV series *Ghost Hunters International*, followed soon after by video horror channel's *Amy's Crypt*. On YouTube I watched the hosts tour the gutted hospital remains. They called the hospital one of the most haunted places in the Philippines, in Asia, perhaps in the world. In 1991 that hospital and all of Clark Air Force Base were buried in volcanic ash from the eruption of Mt. Pinatubo. The base was abandoned.

But I was there in 1959 and my memories of the hospital center on a small bright room surrounding my white-sheeted bed, and a photograph. In the photo I am standing outside in a hospital gown between my two sisters in their Halloween costumes. They teased me that day for being a true skeleton.

A cruel nurse prepped me to take insulin shots by observing me inject into an orange and then into my thigh. She had me fill the syringe with distilled water and I knew it should be saline solution. I suggested that, but she demanded that I inject the water, which hurt and left a red welt.

In accordance with the times, I was directed to inject into my thighs, not into the softer places we use today. Technology was primitive. Insulin is meant to be injected just under the skin, but my needle was long and I often hit muscle—ouch. I had a glass syringe and a stainless steel needle that I sharpened on a whetstone. Both had to be sterilized for every use by boiling for 10 minutes. That long thick needle with jagged edges from less-than-professional sharpening meant injections hurt. I had no fat to inject into. But I was stoic.

My parents had routinely discouraged me from asking for help so at 14 I was already self-sufficient. Over the years I had been turned back to my own resources when seeking help to handle bullies, excessive homework and loss of friends. Therefore, the pronouncement that I had type 1 diabetes didn't deter me. Although my diagnosis was serious and we had no idea what it actually meant, I was relieved to have it named and acknowledged. Lying in my hospital bed after my parents left that first day, I thought, "At least it's something that won't kill me."

Maybe I was an optimist. Certainly my defenses were solidly established. Although my parents maintained a firm foundation for me and my sisters, as military brats we were jerked out of home and school and neighborhood and friendships over and over. We were separated from blood relatives, and forever strangers needing to reestablish ourselves. I learned to distance myself from my emotions.

My war veteran father had piloted a *Flying Fortress* bomber over Germany during World War II. Each morning as he climbed into his B-17 he knew that only half of the planes leaving would return. His beloved older brother, a fighter pilot, was shot out of the sky and killed. I learned these facts from others. Dad did not speak of them. Yet my mother told me he thought my diabetes diagnosis was the worst thing that had ever happened to him. I didn't understand that and we never spoke of it. He was my model. I followed his lead. How could I complain or even show an emotional response to anything less than he had undergone?

Two weeks after my diabetes diagnosis my family and I flew by military transport from the Philippines to our new assignment in California. I was kept in the hospital for those two weeks, not allowed to visit my home or school again. All that I knew from arrival in the Philippines two years before was left behind without a goodbye. Departure in that way at that time seemed even more significant than getting diabetes. There was so much to absorb.

We settled on the central coast of California at Vandenburg Air Force Base. My mother found a diabetes specialist in Santa Barbara and took me there. The presiding MD told me not to eat fruit. And he advised my mother she could oversee every bite I took and every choice I made, or she could give me my freedom. He also quietly told her I might live 10 years. Luckily I had a teen's typical response. I assumed that I would live and do whatever I wanted to do. We never saw that doctor again.

Diabetes altered our family life only somewhat. My mother was both practical and upbeat. She gave me freedom. Home-cooked meals continued, with the addition of side salads. My sisters and I stopped making fudge and made fewer cookies. The bowls of hard candy on our living room table disappeared.

Little else changed with diabetes. I was raised to be independent and was a thinker not a feeler. I mentally worked things through and adopted a serious detached disposition. Diabetes in those days meant one terrible shot a day, taken in the morning and soon left behind. I didn't know about consequences. I didn't know anyone else who had diabetes. I had minimal information so I just went on.

Both of my parents came from poor families and raised themselves up. We had little money but they were thrifty and my father's job was steady. Although we moved every two years, we had a measure of solidity and security because my parents made that for us. The trauma of so much loss and leaving was never addressed.

Mother stayed at home to care for us, and loved art, music and history. When dad was away, she took us to museums and cultural events. She liked to create adventures and told us when setting out for a day of discovery, "Pack your toothbrushes. You never know where we'll end up."

As a military family we lived in California, Florida, Japan, Louisiana, Maryland, the Philippines and South Carolina—adding up to 12 different schools for me before high school graduation. I became adept at quickly finding my way, making friends, and adapting to the surrounding customs. And I did not ask for help.

Preparing for my first new school after diagnosis I decided to paste a smile on my face. For the first few days I staggered around the large campus carrying all my heavy schoolbooks because I didn't understand how to open my locker. Finally a student nearby saw me struggling and showed me how to manage the combination.

Despite diabetes and strict family rules I was never set apart. I had massive opportunity. Although mother stayed at home to take care of us and to be available for my father, she had greater ambitions for her daughters. I became the first person in the history of our family to achieve a college degree.

But when I was diagnosed I was a teenager! Diabetes was not the most important aspect of my existence. I wanted fun with friends, to be on the honor roll, and sometimes to skip school and go to the beach. I joined drama club, Latin club, debate team, and wrote articles for the school newspaper. My friends and I flew screaming over the hills on our bicycles. I learned to drive a car and began dating.

The concept of denial had not yet arrived in social awareness. I did not exactly deny my diabetes, but I held it apart. I took my shots. I ate few sweets. That was mostly all. I certainly did not embrace diabetes, did not talk about or investigate it. I was immersed in completing my junior year in high school and being trained to edit the school newspaper the following year.

Midsummer my father announced that we were moving again. Suddenly we packed up, crowded into our small family car and were driven cross country to a new home in Maryland. The relationships and the life I had established in California were ripped away. That change was the most difficult yet. I was almost grown and had built a world for myself. My beloved Siamese cat was left behind, as was the boldness and individuality of the West. Ahead of me loomed more fixed and traditional terrain. I shut down.

As a teen and my parents' daughter, I had no vote in the move. I begged to stay with friends to finish high school in California. But my rights and opinions were overshadowed by both parents, the military, the Catholic Church, and God. Furious, I turned inward, yearning to be free of all rules. As a typical teen I took out my intense frustration on my family. When not in resentful silence I talked back to my parents and bullied my younger sisters.

The rules of type 1 diabetes care and what might be considered its attendant loss of freedom were not yet apparent. I remember nothing at all about diabetes affecting my life. My senior high school year was unpleasant for other reasons. I knew how to drive but we had only one family car and lived in the suburbs so I could not get a job. My school was not racially integrated. I was uncomfortable with the social attitudes surrounding me. My feature stories for the school newspaper were considered subversive and not printed. I felt imprisoned. In response I was resentful and often bitchy. My boyfriend took me swimming one afternoon and I fussed so fiercely about not getting my curled hair wet that he said, "You're almost as much fun as being with someone."

Finally I graduated high school and left my family home in Maryland to attend Macalester College in St. Paul, Minnesota. I wanted to be a journalist. My parents had pressured me to go to the gigantic University of Florida because my father claimed Florida citizenship and I would qualify for in-state tuition. Instead I secured grants and scholarships to make up the financial difference. Macalester, besides its small size, lack of sororities, and journalism program, was a step west. Mother and dad loved the South and had returned us there as often as possible. But I wanted to go back to the wide-open sense of possibility and independence I had experienced in California.

In college I knew no one with diabetes and continued to receive no guidance for living with it. My college dormitory had a kitchen where I refrigerated my insulin and boiled my glass syringe every morning, then took my daily shot. By that time disposable needles were available, so I didn't have to sharpen and boil my needles. I don't remember talking about my diabetes with anyone. I do remember eating massive sweet rolls drenched in honey from a nearby Greek café, so I was not exactly eating well. Or was I addressing midafternoon NPH hypoglycemia?

I earned average grades and drifted from language study to political science, finally majoring in English. My primary education involved relationships, and whether as an obvious sinner I could continue with Catholicism. My urge for independence, deep and true from early years, greatly helped me arrange my life with type 1 diabetes. But I had no idea who I was. And I had no partnership with my diabetes.

On a weekend retreat to the Chicago Theological Seminary, I was awakened every morning with a gong and a resident calling out, "Christ has risen. So should you." I shared my experiences there with another student whose home was in Durango, Colorado. Her parents were friends with the publishers of the town newspaper. She contacted them for me, and I spent my college senior year internship writing for the *Durango Herald*.

For that month in Durango I flourished as a general assignment reporter, applying my photography and writing skills in features and news stories. The small town surrounded by mountains seemed ideal. The *Herald's* publishers asked me to join their staff as soon as I graduated from Macalester. I did. I stepped west. I never returned to California, but the Rocky Mountains have been my home for all my adult life.

At age 20, living in my little Colorado town, diabetes finally raised its head and challenged me. Hospitalized with an urgent yeast infection, I was soundly warned that my blood sugar was too high. That was my first face-to-face encounter with the threats of type 1. The medical professionals I encountered provided censure and little direction. I still didn't specifically know what to do to take care of myself. Fortunately, circumstances drew me into the mountains. There I was able to hike my blood sugar into control and to build my self-awareness.

How could I create a positive relationship with my diabetes when I finally understood that it could harm me? That would come with time. I didn't know enough about type 1 or about myself, and I needed to find support.

CHAPTER 2

Next Steps to Incorporating Diabetes

*Freedom comes from diving deeply within
and knowing who you truly are.*

Amy Leigh Mercree,
Author and Medical Intuitive

Throughout my life I have chased freedom. As a girl, my favorite song was *Don't Fence Me In*. As a teen I yearned for wide open spaces where I could find myself. Freedom is the reason I moved to an isolated Colorado town of 10,000 residents to become a newspaper reporter.

My daily reporter's beat included taking photographs for the front page, and asking for news at the Sheriff's office and police station. I toured the countryside looking for people and events to write about. I was fearless. When roads were blocked for the filming of *Butch Cassidy and the Sundance Kid,* I trekked through stubbled hayfields to knock on the door of a ranch house. Willing strangers lent me Levi's and boots to wade across the river and sneak onto the film set.

I fished for trout with the proprietor of a rock shop, and his wife taught me to find and cook puffball mushrooms. A rancher helped me bang together a loom with scrap wood from her barn and showed me how to weave Navajo style. I helped the county agent roll his terrifyingly rustic single engine plane out of a barn. He flew me over Telluride, where he dipped a wing to the old men he knew were drinking coffee on the porch of the general store.

Each afternoon I returned to my office at the *Herald* to hurriedly tap out stories on a Royal typewriter and meet my deadline. I lived in the land of my dreams.

Kentucky Fried Chicken dinners were my mainstay, purchased on the way home to my wood-stove-heated cabin with an outhouse. I salivated as I drove into the Animas Valley, stomach growling at the scent of fat and salt and other deliciousness. I most loved the mashed potatoes and gravy so I dove into those two containers first. The only vegetables in my dinners comprised coleslaw—which I despise and would not have eaten. In those days, fresh vegetables were trucked into town only once a week.

But fruit grew everywhere. I made jelly out of chokecherries and crabapples. I bought a pressure cooker and simmered apples into apple butter. I mimicked the Mormon ladies' strawberry pies only available once a year at the county fair. That attempt was never successful.

My life was rich and satisfying. Although I was admitted to

hospital briefly with high blood sugar, my diabetes regimen did not change. T1D remained a silent partner. I still didn't know what I was supposed to do and wasn't getting helpful advice. Although I limited sweets, I ate bread and potatoes and rice without realizing their effect. I had no way to check my blood sugar. I simply injected a high dose of NPH insulin each morning that sent me crashing into hypoglycemia midafternoon. But I made do. That was the diabetes life I knew. Meanwhile I spent my weekends hiking and camping, which led to my next level of freedom.

A year had passed and it was time for me to leave Durango. An unfortunate relationship shattered the joy I had felt living in my little town and pursuing my reporting job. A neighbor who emigrated from Britain to advise the Colorado Outward Bound School swept me onto COBS' first course for females. I gave notice at work and left to backpack, sail and river raft for 28 days with Outward Bound.

That first course was phenomenal. I loved wilderness camping and wanted to live that way forever. So I trained to become an Outward Bound instructor. Over the next 10 years I seasonally mountaineered as a guide for teachers, teenagers, women over 30 and a few men soon to be released from prison who were sent to be socialized. Mountain living kept me healthy as well as bestowing greater confidence and introspection.

But my mountain lifestyle crashed when a September Outward Bound course was snowed out. With three other instructors I camped a few miles into Colorado's Uncompahgre National Forest with teen boys and girls from a rehab center and settled for the night. When we rose at dawn, two feet of snow covered our campsite. The novice campers had scattered boots and packs and jackets and mess kits outside their tents and all of it was buried in snow. We recovered what we could, marched downhill to the road and forestalled hypothermia while waiting for rescue. The students refused to continue, so that course was canceled and we were bussed back to the city.

Devastated by what I considered my inability to hang on to those difficult students, I entered graduate school for a master's degree in teaching. My new plan was to teach English literature to high school students, which demanded that I improve my leadership skills. And personally I needed greater insight to relate more directly with my diabetes.

My interpretation of freedom was shifting. Although I didn't study philosophy or psychology, I had a psychologist as a college counselor and he made me think. I determined that my fate was in *my* hands, and that I both could and had to choose my responses to anything life brought me—including reluctant students and diabetes. I still didn't know enough about caring for my physical health but acknowledging the reality of my type 1 diabetes gave me greater self-understanding. I began thinking of diabetes as my ally, and included that quirky ally in my life plan.

After I completed graduate school I traveled with a lover, married him and moved to Boulder, Colorado. Bicycling around town and hiking in the foothills bolstered my health as I discovered *New Age* therapies. Influential Naropa Institute had just opened in Boulder and was offering Buddhist meditation retreats. I meditated with the Buddhists. Ida Rolf moved there in 1970 to start the Rolf Institute. I met her as a seamstress and altered her clothing while I learned about and signed up for Rolfing. I made friends with all sorts of practitioners and experienced Feldenkrais, Structural Patterning,

Jin Shin Jyutsu and I'm OK/You're OK therapy.

Diabetes rose higher in my consciousness. Although I did not talk with my spouse or friends about it, I knew I needed a health care team. Beginning my search, I visited a series of medical doctors and alternative healers. The MDs told me I had to do better, but provided no helpful suggestions. The healers recommended dietary, physical and mental approaches but knew little about T1D. Letting it all swirl through my consciousness I raised vegetables in a large garden and ran a neighborhood food coop, disappearing periodically to lead wilderness courses.

Continuing to evolve, I realized that my husband and I had very different life agendas. I left my marriage, learned more about my body's needs, and ardently journaled. That's when I discovered Jess Stearns' book *Yoga, Youth & Reincarnation* and decided I had chosen diabetes as a way to shape my destiny.

CHAPTER 3

What's the Point?
Finding a New Frame for Type 1 Diabetes

Establishing a personal philosophy that lasts takes life experience. In those early years I had no idea who I was as a person with diabetes. T1D was a specter, an unknown, a mystery. I was told that it was deadly but I didn't really know how it was affecting me. Taking insulin daily was my only guideline. I let my diabetes be, turning instead to developing into a reliable adult, figuring out how I belonged in the world. I didn't exactly ignore or deny my diabetes. But I had no idea how to incorporate T1D. And I had excellent training in hiding or burying my feelings. So my thoughts and emotions were not aligning with my reality.

My life shifted when I began to believe that every circumstance can be turned into a gift. We interpret what happens to us. And you know people who can turn any circumstance into a tragedy. On television, actors with millions of followers go from disaster to further disaster and viewers are enthralled. When I watch them, I yell at the TV, "Don't fall for that! Walk out the door!" But falling into tragedy feeds the compelling drama. Dipping into another person's drama may be entertaining. Living there yourself may not.

All of us venture into our mudholes sometimes. We can even get upbeat there. *Happy as a pig in mud* is listed in *Merriam-Webster Dictionary* as an idiom for very happy. Kids get happy in mudholes. I remember running barefoot through the flooded ditches in Florida's warm rain when I was five years old. I was wet and muddy and joyous, and I can go there now in my mind. That's the image I seek nowadays when I'm stuck in a mudhole in my good clothes getting surly.

Choosing to call my life good and to find gifts in difficult circumstances—like having type 1 diabetes—works for me. I consider optimism an asset. I may not call my circumstances good immediately. There may be need for a turnaround. But I can get there if I want to. I have the choice. If that isn't your path yet, try it. Build on your attempts until choosing goodness and gratitude becomes a habit.

Consider how your life might change if you framed type 1 diabetes as the best gift you've ever received. Maybe start by considering it merely a neutral intrusion into the life you thought you'd have, and work forward from there.

You might entertain these ideas I adopted from a philosophical webinar I attended:

- Everything about my life has been chosen (by me) for my soul's development.
- Out of the most challenging times comes the greatest transformation.

- Everything that occurs in my life is part of the amazing adventure of my soul.

There are countless ways to instill meaning in your life with diabetes. One that I use almost every day is to accept that I chose diabetes for my soul's development. With that assumption, my search for freedom takes on deeper meaning. The freedom I am seeking is transformation, and diabetes is part of the big adventure leading me there.

Humans continue to evolve, in lifetimes as well as eons. Why not believe that hard times invite us to be stronger and to create a richer future?

You may already have stopped listening to inner or outer voices concentrating on the negative and pulling you down. Instead you choose thoughts and activities that lift you. There are some simple steps you might have taken. Turn off the news. Play music you love. Look out the window. Pet your cat. Walk your dog.

What might you do to lift yourself out of negative thoughts about your diabetes? When it's time to check your blood sugar or inject insulin or change your infusion set, thank your body for all it does for you. Laugh at yourself when you get pissy. Make time for diabetes demands so you aren't rushed and overwhelmed. Create a routine that makes your diabetes care easy. Those are all choices you can accomplish. Success with that and you may take on the impossible—making T1D an asset.

As I think about the power of choosing, three truths come to mind. You may already be considering these. First, it is possible to live a happy life with type 1 diabetes. Second, you are worthy of excellent health. And third, other type 1 humans need you.

First, it is possible.

On my wall is a framed collage I bought years ago. Around a 5-cent postage stamp with the image of an airplane the artist wrote, "It has never been done & it cannot be done. I told Wilbur that. And I told Orville that. And I am telling you that."

I am telling you that anything is possible. Although it seemed impossible, Wilbur and Orville flew. Although it seems impossible, you can flourish with type 1 diabetes. Books and blogs and diabetes communities relate stories of those who have prospered with type 1 diabetes, not in spite of it but *because* of it. Anything is possible for you.

Second, you are worthy.

Thousands of worthiness quotations appear online, including hymns and bible verses. Here are two that express my thoughts.

You are valuable because you exist. Not because of what you do or what you have done, but simply because you are.

Max Lucado
Christian Author & Pastor

Worthy now. Not if. Not when. We are worthy of love and belonging now. Right this minute. As is.

Brené Brown
Author, Researcher, Professor

Just for being human, but perhaps particularly because you are a human who has type 1 diabetes, you are of great value. Although there's nothing you need to accomplish to be of value, I ask you to consider how important it is that you care for yourself physically, emotionally and spiritually. Because...

Third, we need you.

We need each person on our planet to contribute what only they can offer for the good of all of us. With a breath of relief, I join those who think like me and believe what I believe. But I am also served by those most unlike me who cause me to look again at my own values and know more about myself. I am not a hero and you don't have to be a hero. Be your valuable self. Shine in your own way and let goodness spread out from you to support others.

"It is necessary when in darkness to know that there is light, that deep within oneself there is light." Since my college years I have remembered this quote in troubled times and attributed it to James Baldwin. But I have never been able to recover the exact words. Tonight, after meditating, it came to me again. I want myself to know and I want you to know that deep within ourselves there is light. And our light is needed upon this earth. That is why I tell you that you must take care of yourself! Whatever light you bring, humanity needs.

Forgive my musts. But you must discover how best to care for yourself and do it! No matter what's happening in your country, your state, your town or your home, you must take care of yourself. You must find the support you need, the medication you need and the inner fortitude you need to meet anything life brings. You must survive. You may be inspired to work publicly in the highest good of all. Or you may live quietly and seek to know and express yourself in more private ways. Whatever your destiny, take care of yourself. Stay strong. Make type 1 diabetes your ally.

We are worthy of full expression no matter what label is applied to us. Whoever we become and however we choose to express ourselves, we are needed. Good-hearted people are needed. Friends and sisters and brothers and mothers and fathers and loners and extroverts are all needed. With our awareness as type 1s we have valuable thoughts and feelings to share about human experience. Take charge of your health and your beliefs. Partner with your diabetes. Stay strong. Be well, and help us all create the world we want to live in.

PART 2

DIABETES IN YOUR OUTER WORLD

CHAPTER 4

What They Say & What You Know
You Need to Build a Team

Type 1 diabetes is complex and relentless. We will see dozens, maybe hundreds, of medical professionals in our lifetimes and few will be aware how diligently we care for ourselves. Even fewer will be appreciative and uplifting.

In the 1990s, waiting to be seen in my general practitioner's office, I sat with my head down and thought hard about how to explain what was happening with my diabetes. I needed help. His nurse showed me into the antiseptic exam room, decorated only with the doctor's credentials. She weighed me and took my blood pressure, which was high. Finally the doctor came in.

"How are you?" he asked.

"I am going into menopause," I blurted, "and my insulin regimen isn't working anymore."

He interrogated me about my habits, whether I was taking my insulin, whether I was depressed. Then he leaned in so close I could see the stains on his lab coat. He sniffed me and demanded, "Are you drinking heavily? Are you lying to me about what you eat?"

I was stunned. He had sped past my sincere explanations and branded me a liar trying to cover up for bad self-care. I should have pointed my finger at him and shouted. I should have stormed out. I should have complained to someone—but who could I complain to?

Instead I reverted to the good Catholic girl I had been, still the brave little solder raised by my war veteran dad. I held my feelings in. I listened until the doctor was done and left to cry in the parking lot. But I did not schedule a follow-up.

Primary care physicians are most often the medical providers who care for people with both type 1 and type 2 diabetes. They are frequently kind and helpful people. They may be the only docs for many miles in rural areas or the only ones your insurance covers. But they are almost always pressed for time and might lack communication skills. Most important, they may be entirely unable to address the complexities of type 1 diabetes.

That righteous physician who was sure I had lied to him referred me to a diabetes educator, which turned out to be a tremendous favor. But I hated him for his judgments and for making me feel bad and wrong.

I made an appointment with the diabetes educator and marched into her office with my fists clenched.

"I want to harm my doctor," I told her. "I want to burn his house to the ground."

"Well, you can't do that," she declared, "so let's talk."

I talked nonstop in great frustration and she listened. Her office was small so I couldn't pace. Squirming, I insisted I was strictly following my diabetes plan. I was careful with carbohydrates, covered what I ate with insulin and stayed active. I was doing my absolute best, but blood sugar swings were interrupting my sleep. Both highs and lows were keeping me from my work and my relationships. On top of all that, I had the symptoms of menopause. And the doctor who referred me to her had swept right past all that to blame me!

Paula came around her desk to sit beside me and followed every word I said. She nodded and tsk-tsked in agreement. Then she told me it was true that a woman's medication needs might change with menopause. Insulin is a hormone and my hormones were shifting. She determined that I needed a 20% *reduction* in the amount of insulin I was taking. My blood sugar had been rebounding from high to low and back to high, wrecking me emotionally and physically.

How would I have ever figured that out? How could a primary care physician know that? I wept in relief and frustration. And I cried for all the other good-girl or good-boy type 1s who met with unknowing caregivers and might never get respect and useful information.

Paula gave me extra time that day. When she stood to conclude our meeting she declared, "You should be sitting in my chair."

Oh my God! She believed me. She honored me and my experience. She knew how difficult my life had been and that this imbalance wasn't my fault. She interacted with the real me. I stood up straighter, feeling proud, knowing her advice would set me straight and I would be fine. I could not yet imagine myself as a diabetes educator, but I left relieved and hopeful about my health.

Paula's knowledge and attitude opened new doors for me. When her invitation sank in, I decided to become a diabetes educator, and went back to university for a master's degree in health education. I volunteered in the community clinic where I met Paula. And more than 20 years later I still check in with her to update my own diabetes care.

I have seen other excellent diabetes educators as a patient, and my own diabetes education practice is based on those meetings. I want my clients to know that I believe in them. I value their experience and I am on their sides. I want to listen to them, offer real solutions and show my respect.

My demoralizing meeting with that uninformed "Are you lying to me?" doctor was a brief episode in my health history. But biased assumptions about diabetes are too common. Two years ago I was tipped back in an ophthalmologist's treatment chair, prepped for an injection in my right eye for diabetic macular edema. Unsuspecting, I had arrived for a procedure by my usual trustworthy doctor. But he was ill and I was assigned to his substitute. I had never met the doctor filling in for my regular specialist.

Substitute doc marched into the room where I waited nearly upside down and ready for an injection. Looking at my chart and not at me he announced, "You wouldn't be here if you took care of your diabetes."

I was inverted, my right eye filled with anesthetic goo and covered by a patch. And the medical assistant had ordered me to stay still. So I silently cursed that asinine doctor while he injected the drug that would keep my eye safe for two more months. He strode out of the treatment room and disappeared. Reeling as I stood, my poor eye stinging, I walked out of the clinic and sat in my car until I recovered enough to drive home. I changed my eye care to another medical practice.

What might have prevented that experience? I was treated in that clinic regularly and well-known there. Why didn't they warn me, or reschedule me? As you have probably already discovered, medical practices don't want to miss being paid for a procedure. Had I found out about the change that morning when I was checking into the clinic and canceled my appointment, I would have been charged for it. Further, I needed the injection and my regular doctor came in from another city only once a week—so waiting for him meant my eyesight would be threatened. My choices were limited.

Sometimes I do feel victimized. I need ongoing medical assistance yet I am bound by the rules accompanying a certain doctor, clinic, procedure, my insurance or the system itself. The response I have come up with is a kind of prayer. I get calm, thank my body for its resilience, and assure myself that I am cared for on a deeper level than any bad person or bad experience can threaten. Waiting in a clinic for a doctor to arrive, I withdraw into a meditative state and rely on my inner resources. I imagine guardian angels around me who make sure that I am surrounded with light, and guide my providers to do their very best work.

People with type 1 diabetes have been pounded and we are tender. Often diabetes is not our primary problem. The problem is how the outside world responds to our diabetes. We are often criticized and accused of being noncompliant when we are doing all we can but our regimens aren't working. Unlike those with physical conditions like cancer or arthritis, we are regularly blamed for our diabetes. Outsiders assume that if I had eaten better or exercised more or taken the right amount of insulin at the right time or embraced miraculous alternatives, I would be problem-free. The everyday ups and downs of type 1 diabetes are exhausting. Yet we are forced to defend ourselves. We may have little energy to deal with punitive *experts* who are meant to be helping us.

There are helpful steps you can take.

- Find the right medical practitioner.

- Assure that you see who you meant to see, and be an advocate for yourself.

- Take a friend with you.

Excellent advice that I don't always follow.

In 2017 I went to a weekend retreat in San Diego called *One*, sponsored by the Taking Care of Your Diabetes nonprofit. Being in a conference room with hundreds of other T1Ds, with type 1 experts on stage, was exquisite. People had continuous glucose monitors or pods on their arms with patches decorated like tattoos. Pumps and other gear beeped and buzzed. We wore nametags that indicated how long we'd had diabetes. Mine read "LEGEND 30+ years." I was with my people.

One of the breakout sessions was *When Diabetes Gets Complicated*, led by Type 1 blogger and author Kerri Sparling. (You can view that session and others at tcoyd.org.) Kerri opened with her awareness that complications of type 1 diabetes are most often dealt with as something we did wrong. "Guilt is built in," she said, and invited people's stories of good and bad medical encounters.

These comments from the audience particularly resonated for me:

- We don't always get medical checkups because we're afraid of being shamed.

- We saw every single endocrinologist in Orange County and kept firing them. If your physician isn't good for you, ditch 'em and move on.

- I am my own advocate. I listen to the doctors but I have an opinion.

- I was young. I didn't say anything.

- We are supposed to know better.

- The burden of being blamed is part of having diabetes.

- Type 1 takes tremendous courage.

We all have to find our own ways to address poor treatment. And we do need to be courageous. Some of the people commenting during that session called themselves warriors. My strong belief is that if I consider myself a warrior I live at war. I don't want to impose war on myself. I don't want to fight or to confront hidebound providers—especially when I need their help.

When treated badly I have not always reacted in my own best interest. But there are myriad ways to respond. Like Mahatma Gandhi, I am devoted to passive resistance.

You will find your way. Be prepared. Be careful what you believe. There's garbage information on the Internet and there may be garbage information in your doctor's office. Get second opinions. Find medical professionals who appreciate you and can express their warm hearts. T1D is hard enough without judgmental attitudes and pronouncements, and certainly without ignorance that can harm you. Even the greatest expert may have beliefs about your health that are not appropriate for you.

Scientific research indicates that *tight control* reduces the risk of diabetic complications and mortality. Keeping your blood sugar as steady as possible in the 7% or lower A1c zone is supposed to keep you safe. The 1980s Diabetes Control & Complications Trial (DCCT) supposedly *proved* that good control reduced your risk of microvascular complications. However, Steven Edelman, T1D endocrinologist and director of Taking Care of Your Diabetes, revealed in that breakout session that preferential treatment assisted those in DCCT's tight control cohort. He said the trial's successful intensive therapy group was richly supported. They were assigned nurses and doctors and investigators who called them on the phone, met them regularly in the clinic, had them over for dinner and gave them baseball tickets! That successful research group was not handling tight control alone. They had fantastic teams!

Did I need a team? I took care of my condition entirely alone for many years. But I learned the value of support when my diabetes educators championed me. Instead of avoiding the medical world and hacking my way through the jungle of diabetes care alone, I began to gather my experts.

Seeing doctor after doctor, being judged and having to fire them is debilitating. Your health is enhanced and may even be saved with a circle of professionals who are well-informed about your kind of diabetes, and who, most of all, honor and empathize with you. Your team will be different from anyone else's and it will shift to meet your changing needs. Find your team!

CHAPTER 5

Building Your Team

Acknowledging that I needed to create a primo team I began to assemble championship players. My current team includes:

1. Me
2. Primary Care Physician
3. Endocrinologist
4. Diabetes Care & Education Specialist
5. Ophthalmologist + Optometrist
6. Dermatologist
7. Chiropractor/Naturopath
8. Pilates Instructor
9. Spiritual Advisor
10. Family Members & Friends

Notice that I am the team leader! My diabetes health is in my hands. My team provides advice and specific knowledge I don't have. But I decide how to apply their knowledge and advice. And I am the one who must act. Team members augment different aspects of my health. I listen and learn, decide and move forward with what's right for me.

I now have a great **Primary Care Physician** who monitors my overall health and is available to help with emergencies or hospitalization. Dr. Parke laughs with me. She starts our visits sipping her iced coffee and smiling. "You're doing great!" she says, "How can I help?"

Several years ago I underwent surgery for a melanoma that included removal of lymph nodes. I had a primary care physician I didn't know very well and didn't inform her that I was having surgery. When the incision on my thigh became infected after surgery, I urgently requested an appointment with that doctor. She looked at my red and heated wound, shook her head, and referred me back to the surgeon. He handed me over to a scornful assistant who believed I had not followed post-surgery instructions. She sent me home untreated.

It had taken tremendous energy and persistence to even get those two to see me. Neither one provided me with therapy or solace. No one was on my side. I was in pain. My wound throbbed and I knew something was wrong. I felt defeated and betrayed. I was afraid I might go to sleep and not wake up.

Late the following night, really ill by then, I asked a neighbor to take me to the hospital emergency room. Emergency room staff quickly swooped me in, afraid I was going into diabetic ketoacidosis, and I was diagnosed with a staph infection. Fluid under my wound was painfully drained and I lay on a gurney for several hours getting hydrated with intravenous fluids. Then I was ushered out on crutches. For two weeks I could barely walk. I languished in my living room on a borrowed patio chaise longue, surviving on canned soup.

That was the sickest I remember being since my diabetes diagnosis. Worried that I would never recover, I was deeply discouraged and had trouble accepting how vulnerable I was. As I healed, I realized that I needed a physician within the local medical system who would stand with me when I was in trouble and make sure I was properly treated. I needed to take a friend with me to appointments to speak up when I couldn't. I needed to choose a surgeon who was as good with his patients as he was with cutting out skin cancers and lymph nodes. I needed a team that was committed to me.

Now I have a primary care physician who supports my everyday health needs and likes me!

Next on my team is an **Endocrinologist**, who knows the intricacy and the particulars of type 1 diabetes. Unfortunately, many areas have no endocrinologists. In New Mexico there aren't enough endocrinologists to take on the type 1 population. Specialists are periodically flown in from other states to deal with complex patients.

Sources for better care are increasing. Investigate possibilities. You may be able to arrange appointments with an endocrinologist anywhere via telemedicine, internet or phone. Or your local doctor could present your case for feedback through an organization like Project ECHO (Extension for Community Healthcare Outcomes) and learn from an expert. In several states Project ECHO provides isolated or rural providers with access to specialists and academic or medical centers.

Sign up with an endocrinologist if you possibly can and meet with them as often as possible. Even if they are not emotionally supportive, you may benefit greatly from their expertise. But if you have further choice, find one you like! And many endocrinologists have diabetes educators in their offices, or work with one they can refer you to. Take advantage.

My endocrinologist is responsible for prescribing my insulin, insulin pump, continuous glucose monitor and supplies. Besides lab reports she can view statistics and patterns from my insulin pump and continuous glucose monitor on her computer screen. She sees insulin use, carbohydrates covered, time in range, blood sugar highs and lows, all spanning the last 90 days, so she can evaluate and advise with timely information.

I like my endocrinologist and have seen her quarterly for several years. She has learned more about how diabetes works in my body and tailored her care to my situation. The first time I saw her, she asked for my insulin pump and began reprogramming it without explaining what she was doing. She changed my settings to give me the standard 50/50 basal/bolus rate, even though my diabetes educator had set it at 35/65, which better matched my insulin use. The following morning, I woke with blood sugar at 50, and changed my pump settings back.

During our first encounter I hadn't the confidence to tell my endo why my insulin levels were set as they were. And I didn't say a word as I handed her my pump and watched her reprogram it. As was my habit, I deferred to authority, and my ingrained reticence kept me silent. Fortunately, I gained self-assurance and became a better partner in our encounters. Now I feel free to tell her what's important to me.

Remember that you are the team leader! You may need to upgrade your diabetes awareness. You may need to get past your tendency to hold back. Speaking up is vital, because you know more about your own health, habits and goals than anyone else. How can anyone else determine what's right for you unless you tell them?

Essential on my team is my **Diabetes Care & Education Specialist**. She is smart, encouraging and extremely knowledgeable about all aspects of type 1 diabetes. According to the Association of Diabetes Care and Education Specialists:

> As a member of your diabetes care team, a diabetes care and education specialist works with you to develop a management plan that fits your lifestyle, beliefs and culture. They'll help you understand how to use devices like meters, insulin pens, pumps and continuous glucose monitoring devices; and use the information from these devices and your lifestyle to identify patterns and opportunities for improvement. You'll work together to find solutions to address your most pressing challenges.

My next team member became a regular because eye trouble led me to improve my diabetes care in the 1980s. Diabetic retinopathy was building and I didn't realize that until the blood vessels in my eyes began hemorrhaging. My vision became so blurred that I needed to hold onto a friend when we went hiking. If one eye bled and impaired my vision I dared not drive my car anywhere because the other eye might fill with blood while I was away from home, completely blinding and stranding me. My normal activities were curtailed, I felt isolated, helpless and terrified of permanently losing my sight.

The first **Ophthalmologist** I saw immediately lasered me; and over time I went through many more laser treatments to stabilize my retinopathy.

About 15 years ago diabetic macular edema set in. Inflammation and swelling progressed in my right eye and needed ongoing treatment. The specialist who first treated my macular edema lasered me, which did no good. The next doctor ignored my edema. When a new member of his team took over, that doctor clearly explained my worsening situation and possible treatments, and I agreed to injections. Those painful bimonthly injections inserted minute capsules of medications called anti-VEGF drugs. (VEGF stands for vascular endothelial growth factor.)

Injections through the outer layer of my precious right eye worked for edema, but the process took a toll. I had to take a day off work, and the following day at work was not always easy. The actual procedure was uncomfortable and risky. I was forced to sign papers—provided after my eyes were dilated so impossible to read—that excused the doctor and his practice from any liability, and assured that I would pay the outrageous price for the injection if my insurance refused. I had to promise that a companion was available to drive me home, which I lied about. After each procedure I staggered out into the hallway to make another appointment—which they would not allow prior to treatment.

I learned to be more demanding. The first practice that provided this treatment used a gel in my eye to deaden sensation, applied three times. Then my eye was held open with a device that I was sure tore out eyelashes. I was told to look at the ceiling and hold still, and the doctor injected the capsule. The American Academy of Ophthalmology states that the medication is inserted "through a very slender needle" but it felt like a fat sewing needle. I knew that if his hand slipped I could be blinded. And if he injected through a blood vessel, leakage left my eyeball red for days or weeks.

When the doctor I trusted to make those injections retired I changed practices. My current eye specialist is wise and he listens.

For my first injection in the new practice, prep staff skipped the gel and the doctor injected anesthetic directly into my eye. So I had not one but two injections. I fought that decision, found out the name of the gel—which apparently was more expensive than the injected anesthetic, and had to be specially ordered for me. It was made available, and for my second injection the assistant who applied the gel didn't administer it the way I remembered, so I called for her supervisor. He muttered his way through an explanation but finally took over.

Over several years I worked through all the anti-VEGF drugs available for bimonthly injections and they began to have diminished effectiveness. In 2019 I agreed to an implanted steroid capsule that is said to control edema for about two years—a great relief. I was assured that the level of steroids would not affect my blood sugar, which it has not. My steady eyesight has made every minute of apprehension worthwhile. After 16 months small cysts appeared and I needed a booster of one of the shorter-term anti-VEGF drugs. Although that was unexpected, I confirmed with another specialist that it is not unusual.

My general eye health is overseen by a **Doctor of Optometry**. The original optometrist who diagnosed my glaucoma had a staff that did not welcome me. And his employee choices seemed to get worse.

At my final visit to his clinic the person testing my vision said she had been hired to tattoo eye liner and eyebrows. I was not pleased that the medical assistant evaluating my vision before I saw the doctor was primarily trained in cosmetics. When another young woman ushered me into an exam room and heard me tell the doctor why I had not continued his suggested protocol, she hissed "noncompliant" as she slithered out the door. I stopped going to that clinic.

Next on my team is my **Dermatologist** who does a full-body scan quarterly. As a pale-skinned Anglo who lived in the tropics as a child and at high altitude as an adult, I have had five melanomas that needed surgery. Those too are life-threatening! Remember that you are a human being with health challenges that are not all connected with diabetes. Get everything checked.

Teams are adjusted to meet our needs. At times my team has included a dietitian, podiatrist, hearing specialist, gynecologist, physical therapist, psychologist, massage therapist, and others.

My quality of life has been enhanced by a broad spectrum of alternative therapies. My current **Chiropractor/Naturopath** has significant training in nutrition and uses muscle testing (applied kinesiology) to determine exactly what my body needs. He asks a question about a physical concern or treatment. Then he pushes on my outstretched arm for a positive or negative response. When my arm stays strong and he can't move it, the response is positive.

My **Pilates Instructor** reminds me to stand up straight and tune in to my body. "How does that feel?" she asks me after I stretch or push or pull under her direction. I have to get physical and find out, which is not my usual approach. I do feel better overall when our sessions are complete. "Take it easy and drink lots of water," she advises as I walk out her door.

Curiosity has taken me to both excellent and questionable healers over the years. Most of them have been helpful and a few have not. I once met with a faith healer who taught me to tie my shoes differently so I wouldn't block energy!

A macrobiotic healer insisted that I restrict water and taught me to swallow my pills with a bite of food. Swallowing pills with food is helpful, it pushes down the big ones like fish oil capsules. But not drinking water has become a problem.

A traditional German-born herbalist who ran a store in Boulder, Colorado in the 1970s taught me to make a number of herbal potions, including a hearty lentil soup for vitamin and mineral deficiency.

Unfortunately, I have found that alternative practitioners may be as unaware and judgmental as medical ones. I spoke at a health fair in Tucson, Arizona years ago and wandered around meeting healers at their booths. When I invited one naturopath to attend my talk and learn more about diabetes he snorted and said, "So, you haven't healed yourself!"

A minister or other **Spiritual Advisor** is among those I add to my team. True self-care goes far beyond the physical. Spiritual beliefs and practices are fundamental to my health and happiness. What I believe about life and myself guides my behavior as well as my thoughts. I know that I am a child of God. That makes me worthy of health and happiness. It also gives me reason to take care of myself. I pray. I trust in a source of goodness that is available to all of us. I trust that I deserve comprehensive loving care. I draw that care to me through my team. My team members' appreciation strengthens me, helping me be my healthiest self on all levels.

Family Members and Friends are primary on our teams for most of us. I recommend that you teach your personal team members what you require so they can provide the kind of support you need. In one of the communities where I have worked, people hide their diabetes, even from their families. Failing to alert the people you share your home with about hypoglycemia and how to treat it, for example, may result in unnecessary 911 calls and an ambulance ride to the hospital. I am not willing to take that risk. I have taught my friends to recognize my signs of hypo and to aid me. They sit me down and make me drink juice or eat one of the fruit strips I carry with me.

Family and cultural mores have influenced my health beliefs and behavior. My family taught me to look outside myself for guidance, and for what was considered right or wrong. My primary purpose in this life has been to find out more about myself and to become my own authority. Type 1 diabetes has been my ally in that search.

My diabetes gives me reason to turn inward and become both self-aware and brave. It is difficult even to survive as a person with type 1 diabetes without building capability, awareness and willingness to speak up. How much better could I learn about myself than to have one authority after another question how I handle my diabetes?

For my overall health, I keep track of what medical science recommends, consult with my team, and then decide how to incorporate those possibilities. I have to believe in myself. I believe we have ultimate choice in our lives and ourselves, as we do with our health.

Knowledge about diabetes, and technology, are changing fast.

Find out what can help you live a long and beautiful life. Keep asking questions. The ideal is to live a healthy life with type 1 diabetes—in your own way. You can apply the overarching rules and shape them to fit your life. And you can convene an expert team to enhance your own awareness. It's a tango, not a war.

How might you find your ideal team members?

Make a list of everything important about how you will be treated. Be practical too. You may need to compromise. For example, although I want providers who are kind and good communicators, I chose the best surgeon available for one procedure even though he had no social skills. I knew other members of my team would provide the support I needed. Consider your options case by case. In another instance I chose the better surgeon and that did not work out so well. You learn! Quiz potential team members, watch them, find out about them! Use your detective skills to evaluate them. Notice how you feel when anticipating a visit, during and after.

Some possible considerations:

- Is this person the best at what they do?
- Does this person believe in you?
- Will they interact positively with you?
- Are you treated well by their front office staff and assistants?
- Will they stand up for you (with difficult recovery or insurance claims or other providers) if necessary?
- Will they enhance your health and your life?
- Are they flexible and willing to learn from you?

- What will their practice do if the provider you chose is unavailable?

- Is your provider accessible for between-visit calls or emails?

- Does your health plan cover their services? If not and you still want them, might they join your plan or charge you a lesser fee?

CHAPTER 6

True or False?
Myths & Misunderstandings

What's true about type 1 diabetes and those of us who have it? What's assumed and may be both wrong and held against us? Of the numerous myths and misunderstandings about type 1 that have come my way, these are the ones I bump into most often.

1. What's the big deal? All you have to do is follow a doctor's advice.

2. Anyone can do it, why are you having trouble?

3. There is a strict diabetic diet. You can't eat any sugar or fruit, in fact you should avoid all carbs.

4. Your blood sugar should be 100 mg/dL (exactly and always).

5. When you have to check your blood sugar a lot or take extra insulin you are out of control. You must be doing something wrong.

6. If you do the right things (or eat the right things or follow a certain regimen) you can heal your diabetes.

7. Isn't it wonderful how technology does it all for you? Your pump handles your diabetes automatically, right?

Quick answers first:

1. Doing well with type 1 diabetes *is* a big deal. The advice of a doctor unfamiliar with type 1 may even harm you. Your care is best individualized and overseen by a specialist. Even with such guidance, it's all in your hands.

2. No one can balance type 1 diabetes perfectly. Our bodies are complex and our lives are often unpredictable. Even when we do everything right, things can go wrong.

3. There is no diabetic diet. Type 1s can eat anything. Some choices are better than others. And maintaining a healthy A1c depends on limiting the foods that raise blood sugar.

4. My blood sugar fluctuates regularly. I know the recommended ranges for fasting and after meals and I keep track.

5. Checking my blood sugar often and taking insulin when my blood sugar goes high or when I eat carbohydrates keeps me in good control. Monitoring my blood sugar regularly is essential.

6. At this time, we know of no cure for type 1 diabetes.

7. I handle my diabetes. Technology is helpful, but it
    must be properly set up and regularly evaluated.
    It doesn't always work! My insulin pump is a small
    computer that needs to be programmed and often
    reprogrammed for my needs.

Type 1 diabetes demands an all-encompassing 24/7 lifetime
commitment to your health. There are several fundamental elements
necessary for your survival.

- You need access to insulin.

- You need a knowledgeable primary care physician and
  ideally an endocrinologist.

- You can benefit greatly from a wise and
  compassionate diabetes educator.

- You need personal as well as professional support,
  whether from someone you love or from loving
  yourself.

- You need competency with your insulin basal rate,
  carb coverage and blood sugar testing.

- Attitude counts.

Most essential after insulin is your own attitude. Your medical
provider may not know enough about type 1. You may not have the
best food available. You may not have an insulin pump or a continuous glucose monitor. Those are not essential. You can live well with a
syringe and a vial of insulin. But you must have the will within you
to pay attention, to learn and to do what keeps you healthy.

Life with diabetes isn't either/or. It isn't heaven/hell or good/evil. It's what you choose to do this day, this moment, that sustains or detracts from your health and happiness. And it's also how quickly you recover from unhealthy thoughts or behaviors.

For myself, some days I am perfection. My blood sugar advances steadily in the low 100s. I walk. I eat well. I love myself and I love the whole world. No one else's bad mood affects me. Speeders may cut me off on the highway. My boss may be on a tear. I don't care. I am not limited by the need to check my blood sugar, count carbs and take insulin. I am happy to be alive. All is well.

On other days I am resistant stubborn fury and I hate having diabetes. I eat what I shouldn't, watch TV and play computer games on my couch, repeatedly correct high blood sugar spikes and let opportunity slide by. Everything pisses me off and I yell at my beloved cats. That afternoon or that evening or next morning I recover and start over. I call those days just being human, and I do my best to limit them.

Along my path with type 1 over the years, I have claimed my freedom and lived my life my way. With support from family, friends and professionals, I have taken care of myself. I have a vast array of choices and my choices matter. I am the one who can and who must choose. Some days choosing what's best feels impossible. But for the most part I am in line with my health. I choose again and again what serves me best. Or not. You must choose again and again what serves you best. Or not. This is very clear with type 1 diabetes.

You can imagine why I might have to reach deep for empathy when my type 2 patients tell me they feel fine with their blood sugar in the 300s or 400s; that they can't tell their spouse or mother or daughter how to cook for them; that they don't want to take medications and will improve their lifestyles (but can't and don't). Poking fingers to test blood sugar hurts and besides that the results may be discouraging—so they don't test. Many have told me they hate needles so will never take insulin. (About 50% of type 2s will need to inject insulin after years of diabetes, because their pancreases wear out and stop producing insulin.) I listen and empathize because each of us has places we don't want to go. And although I believe strongly that we all can and must evolve, I know that changing habits is usually hard.

Type 1 is more direct than type 2. I feel definite effects when my blood sugar climbs out of range. My eyes blur and my legs get heavy. My breathing changes. I slow down and my mood plummets. I know then to check both blood sugar and ketones and to take recovery steps.

And even when my blood sugar is perfect I am reminded of my vulnerability. I have pits on the sides of my fingers from years of blood sugar testing, and lumps from thousands of shots. Yet I am grateful that lancets and insulin needles have gotten so short and fine.

But I know type 1s who haven't made peace with their diabetes. Or they have established an uneasy truce after upsetting complications. I camped out with my friend Brian, a single father with two growing children who wanted his children to stay well but forgot himself. His A1c was 10. And my friend Clarice found type 1 so debilitating that she ignored it entirely until Charcot Foot wouldn't even let her walk. We all must choose. And I must deal with the judge in me and trust that we are all doing the best we can.

Because—how well we choose depends. As with so many aspects

of diabetes, we respond to the attitudes of our times and our cultures, and to the demands of our loved ones. Our thoughts and actions are shaped by characteristics and experiences including age, upbringing, economics, friends, where we live, who depends on us and whether we are part of a community with goals that match ours. Economic realities, access to care and our race or ethnic group may help or hinder our ability to reach health goals. In communities where I have worked, people tell me they can't go walking because the neighbors will think they can't afford to drive. Or weight loss may seem impossible in cultures where obesity means you can afford to eat and being thin means you might be starving.

When I was first training to become a diabetes educator, I was firmly advising better nutrition for a male patient with sores on his legs. My mentor pulled me away and whispered that this man stocked shelves in a grocery store and had several children. He fed his family and then ate a dozen corn tortillas to staunch his own hunger. He was paying for his last baby's birth and could not afford medication. I was devastated at my stupidity and have never forgotten that event. That man had his priorities in order. Thankfully, my clinic provided his medication without cost.

Think about how free you have been to choose a particular way of life. Has adjusting for diabetes been difficult? I know that many people with diabetes feel set apart. I thank my mother and father for not allowing that in our family.

There are so many components you have to bring together to build your healthy lifestyles. As John Lennon said, "Life is what happens while you are busy making other plans." No wonder you twitch and fret and lose sleep worrying. Sometimes you won't know what's right or wrong until you try it. And your needs or new habits may confuse or alienate loved ones. When I was newly diagnosed with type 1 and my mother didn't recognize severe hypoglycemia, she slapped me to a stop when I walked out our front door and down the sidewalk in my nightgown.

Even though I have learned a great deal about diabetes and about myself since then, a verbal slap may still knock me off course. Besides handling the 24/7 convolutions of blood sugar, moods, and just dealing with life, I have to respond to everyone else. On one of those days, "Forget it," I spit out, "The rest of you can go to hell."

How is diabetes my ally here? I have had to become more understanding of myself and others. I have had to become a better communicator. Once I recover from a foolish statement aimed at me, I have the opportunity to identify my emotions, clarify my thinking and determine what I really want from a situation. I learn more about myself and what matters to me.

Good communication skills are helpful, and lack of communication can intensify misunderstandings.

When I was growing up my family didn't share how we were feeling, or try to articulate what we were going through. I was trained to be kind and helpful to others, and discouraged from being confrontational—which actually meant not sharing emotions or expressing ideas that might offend anyone else. It was best to keep challenges to myself and deal with them on my own.

That early training has been helpful. But it has its limitations, and I have lost relationships because I didn't speak up about a misunderstanding. Over time I have gained ground in recognizing my emotions, seeing them as mine alone and fleeting. I can usually explain without antagonism nowadays—to come closer to someone rather than push them away.

Here's how I handled one recent experience.

Cottonwood leaves rustled in the wind and were just turning yellow at the end of September on my favorite path along the river. We walked the main trail in our Covid-19 masks and stopped at a bench in the shade, talking amiably. My pump beeped and I slipped it off my waistband to read the message.

"Were you bad?" Ava asked.

"I wasn't bad," I replied, and programmed in a little more insulin. Factually, unemotionally, I told her my endo and I were working to establish better carb coverage. She didn't know what that meant and I did not explain further. We continued our prior conversation. Although I didn't admit a reaction, Ava's remark was engraved on my mind, and I woke in the middle of the night hurt and furious. Was I BAD? Hell no.

Giving up on sleep I got out of bed, turned on the lights, looked at my CGM tracking for the last 12 hours and saw the blood sugar ups and downs that so regularly appear. Why didn't I show her the swings my blood sugar takes? Why didn't I say, "Wait a minute! What brought that on?"

Ava often tells me how impressed she is with all that I do to care for myself as a person with type 1 diabetes. But out of her mouth, unbidden, popped a perfect example of one of the devastating myths we face—attending to insulin or blood sugar meant I had done wrong. She didn't know what my pump beep signaled, but assumed it was a reaction to bad management, and I didn't explain.

Two days later, after working through my emotions and carefully crafting a message, I emailed Ava. I repeated what I had heard her say and asked, "Please tell me anything you can remember about what was behind that question." I thanked her and told her I loved her.

She replied, "I am so sorry, I have absolutely no memory of that nor can I imagine why I would have said that."

Judgmental comments may unexpectedly emerge from anyone we meet. Most people don't know what it's like trying to inject the right amount of insulin to keep blood sugar steady. Or, that a beep from my pump is informational, not a condemnation. It is simply not understood why I have to pay attention to physical changes moment to moment, especially now that I have interactive technology.

But what good would it do for me to stay hurt and angry and not share what I'm going through with a friend? I have never sat down and told Ava or any other friend exactly what a day is like for me. They don't know that I look at my CGM receiver to check my blood sugar 50 times a day and that my pump or CGM beep or buzz me constantly. Every bite I eat is first evaluated. And to get to that hiking spot I had so much more than shoes and hat and lip balm to pull together. Before leaving home my insulin pump, my CGM monitor and my hearing aids had to be charged and I needed to have them all attached to me! My blood sugar had to be in range for driving and then hiking—which meant insulin adjustments or additional food or drink. The reservoir in my pump had to have enough units of insulin. I needed to take sweets with me in case my blood sugar went too low! I had to wear slacks with a solid waistband so my pump wouldn't pull them down. That's my basic prep with current technology. Preparing for an all-day hike is more like gearing up for an expedition.

Here's the key for people who don't have type 1 diabetes. We need insulin for any number of obvious or subtle reasons and our bodies may behave mysteriously. Like people with broken bones who can feel a weather change, our bodies react to everything. I may not eat for hours but my blood sugar rises anyway. Anticipating a potentially stressful event may trigger blood sugar changes. Emotional upheaval may trigger blood sugar changes. And even when I direct my pump to make a correction, that doesn't always solve the problem.

Insulin is a hormone and responds to other hormones in our systems. We can never inject manufactured insulin at the right time or in the right volume for it to work as perfectly as a nondiabetic body automatically does. It is always a crapshoot! *Merriam-Webster Dictionary* defines crapshoot as something that has an unpredictable outcome. That is life with type 1 diabetes.

PART 3

DIABETES IN YOUR INNER WORLD

CHAPTER 7

Depression, Distress or Real Life with T1D?

Another myth you may have bumped up against is the assumption that because you have diabetes you are likely to be depressed. Depression has long been linked with all types of diabetes and may affect you.

Clinical depression is considered a mental health disorder. If you are depressed, or think you might be, talk about your worries with your medical doctor and find a way to meet with a licensed counselor or psychologist. People with depression have found help in therapies of many kinds, and sometimes with medication. Therapy is a valuable opportunity not only to address troubles but to better understand yourself. Getting support from a professional who knows depression and what to do about it is essential.

Meanwhile—all of us have emotional responses to life difficulties, and a number of those are associated with diabetes self-care. A lesser-known diagnosis to investigate is *Diabetes Distress*. The

Society of Behavioral Medicine has a definition: *Diabetes distress is an emotional response to the burdens of living with diabetes and the self-care necessary to manage diabetes.*

How do you know whether you are depressed, distressed, or simply troubled by all that life is currently asking of you? Even mental health experts may find it difficult to differentiate between clinical depression and normal reactions to challenging situations. In the intense extended Covid-19 epidemic and 2020/2021 U.S. election turmoil for example, many of us lost friends and family members, lost trust in our leaders, wondered what to believe and had no idea where our lives would take us. Everything shifted.

While losing loved ones and fearing for our own health, we faced the terrible consequences of violence, overt racism, unemployment, isolation and income loss. Meanwhile people with diabetes were warned that to avoid being at greater risk for Covid-19, we had to keep our diabetes in control.

During that time stress had bad effects on my blood sugar as well as my thoughts. I kept in touch with loved ones and poured myself into my writing. Desperately searching for hope and peace and positivity, I often fell asleep listening to comforting podcasts. Life was extra hard for a while, and perhaps having diabetes seemed harder.

When I thought about what to include in this book, I knew I had to mention depression. But I didn't know much about diabetes distress. I hadn't heard the doctors or the diabetes educators I work with mention it. Therefore, I don't believe this concept is broadly recognized. Looking into diabetes distress, I found that the term was created in 1995 and has gained notoriety because international research suggests that diabetes distress is common and may be a barrier to emotional well-being, self-care and management of diabetes.

Diabetes distress is not a mental illness. And it appears much more frequently than clinical depression among people with diabetes. Recent literature reviews suggest that 30 to 40 percent of adults with diabetes (type 1 and type 2) are likely to report significant levels of diabetes distress over time.

The 2011 second Diabetes Attitudes, Wishes and Needs Study (DAWN2), reported that 14% of its type 2 participants were likely to have depression, but 45% had experienced diabetes-related distress. And few of DAWN2's health care team members asked how diabetes affected participants' lives.

Why isn't anyone talking about this? Why did doctors in a study directed at the wishes and needs of people with diabetes not ask how they felt about their diabetes care?

My doctors don't ask me how diabetes is affecting my life. And I have not always directly asked my clients how diabetes influences their lives. Why aren't we asking that? I even wondered whether it was important to include diabetes distress in my book. But once I began researching this topic I was consumed by it. I needed to know more.

- Is diabetes distress common in people with type 1?

- Is it constant or intermittent?

- If distress is an emotional response to the burdens of living with diabetes—how might we choose better responses?

Searching for clues I found that diabetes distress is acknowledged by numerous influential organizations including the Behavioral Diabetes Institute, whose principals invented the Diabetes Distress Scale; the Association for Diabetes Care & Education Specialists; the Juvenile Diabetes Research Foundation and the Centers for Disease Control. Those four and many other sources offer patient handouts and tips for dealing with diabetes distress.

While I wondered how diabetes distress actually strikes and what to write about it, my own diabetes went briefly haywire.

About 3 p.m. Saturday, I replaced my pump infusion set and insulin cartridge as I do every three days. The pump always ends that task with the warning, "Test BG in 1-2 hours." Because I have limited blood glucose strips, and because I trust my CGM and state-of-the-art pump, ordinarily I do not check my blood sugar in 1-2 hours. I don't even think about it.

That evening after dinner I looked at my CGM and saw a BG of 150. Seemed fine so I went to sleep. But overnight I was awakened several times by insulin pump and CGM alarms. First my BG was high, so I instructed my pump to deliver the suggested bolus and went back to sleep. Later, the *urgent low* signal blasted me. With blood sugar at 20 I staggered into my kitchen, grabbed apple juice and chugged it down. I hoped I wouldn't die. Then I hobbled back to bed and collapsed into sleep. Near dawn the pump sounded a warning again and I woke to discover blood sugar at 300 and rising fast.

That Sunday morning I had anticipated a Zoom visit with a faraway friend. But I was exhausted and now my pump message read *insulin delivery stopped*. I called pump tech support and under the rep's direction reviewed all the alerts I had received overnight.

Needing glasses and more awareness than I had when only half awake, I hadn't read the details.

Scrutinizing messages, I saw that my insulin delivery had stopped and restarted during the night, which the rep warned me meant the infusion set inserted the day before was not delivering insulin properly. (Those of you who wear insulin pumps know that once in a while when you inject a new infusion set it doesn't go in straight and therefore interferes with insulin delivery. That's why they tell you to check your blood sugar in 1-2 hours.)

Reviewing details of warnings through the night, I started to blame myself. "I should have realized. I should have known. I should have gotten up, turned on the lights, found a magnifier, changed my infusion set. I should've…."

Processing all that information under the tech rep's direction I inserted a new infusion set. Then I signed out of tech support and, though distracted, met with my friend. I explained what was going on while responding to further pump and CGM signals.

Zoom conversation over, it was midday, almost 24 hours after changing my gear, and despite the new infusion set, my blood sugar rose to 400 and kept ascending. I was nauseated, achy and stiff-limbed. When the pump repeated the *insulin delivery stopped* message I took an insulin injection with a syringe and dialed tech support again.

After a 45-minute wait, the second rep answered and determined that the problem was with the insulin cartridge I had replaced the day before. I thanked him and hung up cursing. I was no longer blaming myself, just impatient, disappointed and angry about the whole experience. I changed the insulin cartridge, very aware that costly insulin and supplies had been wasted. Three infusion sets, two cartridges and many hours later I was in the 300s and coming down at last.

Although equipment failure was the reason for my troubles, I lost sleep, spent valuable time addressing blood sugar ups and downs, worried about replacing my equipment and insulin, pierced my abdomen and fingertips several times, thought I might die, and blamed myself. Meanwhile I worried about what those dramatic blood sugar *excursions* were doing to my vulnerable eyes, kidneys and blood vessels. Had I experienced diabetes distress? Certainly.

Trying to stay sane and in-charge as I was pounded by blood sugar vagaries and diabetes demands, I hadn't investigated my emotional responses. But immediately afterwards I recognized my distress, acknowledged myself for staying with the process until my dilemma was resolved, and moved on.

Perhaps you have undergone a similar diabetes upset that you can bring to mind.

- How long did you stay there?

- Did you come through unscathed?

- Did you blame yourself?

- How might you dance more skillfully through another diabetes predicament and the feelings that arise?

Without a positive philosophy about yourself and T1D, you might remain disheartened for days. You might even step out of the dance and give up your good care, for a while or forever. There is always choice. Please make choosing the healthy path a given, because you will meet up with distressing circumstances again and again. And your type 1 diabetes tango partner will regularly challenge you to learn new steps.

Even though I don't think diabetes distress is constant for type 1s, there are times when it sweeps you away. Like a passing thunderstorm, diabetes distress unexpectedly crashes in on you—particularly when other stresses are high. Both life experience and technology periodically fail. Type 1 know-how does not always stop things from falling apart. It doesn't matter how long you have had diabetes. Things go wrong. You may go wrong. And high-tech equipment goes wrong. Your phone, your car and your computer have malfunctioned. So will your diabetes gear. Technological treasures don't always work.

Keep dancing! It may help you to know and accept that T1D thunderstorms will strike. When that happens, what's the best road to take? Get over any blame, do what's needed and appreciate yourself even more for all you put up with!

Diabetes distress could be considered a *normal* response for people with a challenging ongoing physical condition. Sinking into diabetes distress is entirely understandable. But staying there is associated with both poor self-care and poor quality of life. You are best served by getting through it ASAP.

Just realizing that you must deal with diabetes distress could be a powerful incentive to continue taking care of yourself. You can also help all of us by teaching your medical team about diabetes distress and how you have dealt with it.

Our medical providers should be more aware of this vital truth for living with type 1 diabetes—that even though experienced, in control and on alert, you may get blindsided. You may falter and your state-of-the-art technological help may give up on you.

Plus, you are not alone. Diabetes distress affects your loved ones too. You may struggle with your own care, but imagine how hard it must be for those who love you to share in your upsets. Parents of children with type 1 particularly must experience diabetes distress as they guide them through T1D thunderstorms. Although I was a teen when diagnosed and my father was a World War II combat veteran, my mother told me he thought my diabetes was the worst thing he'd ever faced.

Is T1D the worst thing you have ever faced? My answer is no. My T1D is challenging, but it's manageable. Other life experiences have seemed worse.

Depression or Distress?

When I came back to the medical world 30 years ago, after trying to handle my diabetes alone, my new physician asked if I was depressed. I replied caustically, "Of course I'm depressed. Wouldn't you be?"

He didn't answer that question, but he referred me to a psychologist. After I completed a series of tests, the psychologist determined that I was not clinically depressed, which pissed me off. I thought I was indeed depressed by all that I was supposed to be doing for my very existence as a T1D, and that the world around me failed to acknowledge the scope of my type 1 demands. But that was not considered depression, and I did not have a name for what it actually was.

Diabetes distress, although not yet fully understood or adopted, is rising in general awareness. As part of the American Diabetes Association's (ADA's) current Standards of Care, medical providers are encouraged to include evaluation and monitoring of diabetes distress as part of diabetes patient care. Further, they are encouraged to provide patients with support and recommendations. Taking action is considered necessary because diabetes distress is reported to negatively affect our well-being and our ability to take care of ourselves.

The ADA actually asks MDs to screen patients for *both* depression and diabetes distress, but they usually miss distress. I experienced the difference just this week when I met with my primary care physician. Her medical assistant evaluated me for depression as she prepped me.

She asked:
- During the last month have you often been feeling down, depressed or hopeless?

- During the last month have you often been bothered by having little interest or pleasure in doing things?

Although I might answer yes to both of those based on what a month is like with T1D, I answered a truthful "No." And I asked her, "What about diabetes distress?" She ignored me and went on with her evaluation.

But a savvy provider might ask:
- Can you tell me one thing about diabetes that has been driving you crazy?

That question I can wholeheartedly answer. It indicates that my medical provider knows I am facing challenges. Ideally she or he will balance the results of my lab tests with my level of diabetes distress. Because, as diabetesdistress.org notes: *How you feel about your diabetes is as important as your glucose numbers or your A1C.*

You need to know what is considered distressful and find out how that affects you. And you may need to enlighten medical professionals. Most health clinics have not acknowledged the importance of asking directly about your diabetes life. If your provider doesn't ask how T1D is affecting you, speak up. Help him or her understand how dealing with T1D affects your overall health and your quality of life. And request assistance if your daily tasks are too much to bear.

Especially if you determine that your level of diabetes distress is high or constant, your life depends on having a frank discussion with members of your health care team. Find out how much they understand and what they recommend. It's not fair that once more you have to be an educator, but often T1D life experience makes you the smartest person in the room.

I hope the entire world will understand how difficult it is to do all that is necessary to prosper with T1D. May parents and spouses and siblings and bosses and best friends and physical therapists and life coaches and all of us be aware of diabetes distress and how to help type 1s address it. May they love and honor us even more because we are humans living with T1D.

If diabetes distress is affecting you, find an MD or diabetes educator or mental health specialist who will help you figure out exactly what you need to do and admire you for doing it.

Aren't Sure? Take the Quiz

There are several measures for diabetes distress, but the Type I Diabetes Distress Scale (T1-DDS) is specific to our circumstances. You can take the T1—DDS quiz for free at diabetesdistress.org. Taking this quiz will help you find out more about yourself and the way you handle T1D disturbances.

Looking at the quiz after my briefly-falling-apart scenario, I found that Item #1 is: *Feeling that I am not as skilled at managing diabetes as I should be.* I did contend with that feeling, but moved past it and hope you will too.

Once you discover how distressed you are, what can you do about it? The Association of Diabetes Care and Education Specialists recommends these basics for responding to diabetes distress:

- seek support
- move your body
- think positive, and
- be good to yourself

That advice sustains me. On diabetes distress days I call a friend, take a walk, read poetry, drink my favorite tea, and let difficult things on my to-do list wait. I may also listen to a spiritual teacher or a motivational speaker and remember all that is good about my life.

It might be helpful to keep a list or even a sticky note on the fridge reminding you what to do when overwhelmed by T1D, because it can be hard to remember when you are in distress.

Members of your health care team should help you find more choices if your own efforts are not enough. Medical providers are advised to refer their patients with diabetes distress to structured educational programs, emotion-focused or cognitive behavioral therapies, or support groups, and to get them on insulin pumps and continuous glucose monitors. (Pumps and CGMs are supposed to simplify our lives—which you know is not always true.)

Find a Support Group

Support groups may be sponsored by your local medical clinic, and are also available online by way of reputable diabetes websites. My friend Della gained confidence as well as valuable information from her online contacts when she was diagnosed with T1D at age 18. Her cohort communicated thoughts on everything she wanted to know about living with her diabetes, especially physical activity, dietary choices and sexuality. She was greatly relieved to have a circle of people like herself to interact with, and to find out they had struggled with their diabetes too. Their companionship provided context as well as reinforcement.

Belonging to a support group may lift you out of distress whether or not the group is specific to type 1 diabetes. Most of us joined or created personal support groups to get through the isolating Covid-19 times. My Mastermind writing group, for example, has helped me through numerous could-have-been traumas. On Mondays we met by Zoom, wrote together and broke into small groups to listen and be heard. Those meetings started my week with optimism and intention. And I embrace podcasts, TED Talks, webinars, meditation training, even kids' books to feel better and encourage myself.

Any outreach that helps us better know and love ourselves is precious. The journal *Patient Education and Counseling* reported on a 2017 study that determined: "Helping T1Ds to become more aware, less judgmental and less reactive behaviorally to what they feel about diabetes and its management may reduce diabetes distress."

All of us *need* ongoing support—from family, friends, providers, educators and most of all from ourselves. And we should never be blamed or expected to blame ourselves for diabetes difficulties.

What if it's just life?

Of course, life distress and diabetes distress intertwine. With or without type 1, life is sporadically hard. However, it is not necessary to endure unrelenting stress or diabetes distress.

How do you maintain your diabetes self-care in the midst of whatever you're going through? How do you remember to care for yourself no matter what? Even if you get help, you must figure it out for yourself. Nothing works for everyone. You adopt an approach, experiment, learn and keep trying. Survival with diabetes becomes second nature. You determine how to get around, through or past diabetes distress. You start over every single moment. It's possible. Living at the edge of death as we do creates perspective and resiliency, and demands courage. But you know that because you are reading this book.

When life is distressful because of T1D or for any other reason, keep your attention on the basics. Do what's necessary to maintain or re-establish healthy blood sugar. Stay wise about your diabetes care as life stresses come and go.

In the midst of big life trouble myself, when tax forms litter my floor and my sister's medical team calls to say she's fallen again, I find working out, cooking, even brushing my teeth impossible. My home needs cleaning, I am eating potato chips instead of dinner, and sleep is tumultuous. My mind insists there's nothing good ahead and

I am not handling my responsibilities well. But I still respond when my CGM beeps and my pump warns me it's running out of insulin. I know my priorities. My type 1 care is essential to my existence. And your type 1 care is essential to your existence.

Some people give up. Their critical thoughts recirculate, "I can't do it. I'm not perfect. Whatever I do won't make a difference. I am a victim to this wretched disease. How can I do all I'm supposed to and have a life? I have no support. I don't know what to do!"

Please don't give up. This book is meant to remind you that type 1 can be the very reason you choose to be fully human. Show others how hard it is and that it's worth it. Become an advocate for yourself and even for the value of having T1D. It is part of everything about your life. While you experience certain aspects of diabetes that might be considered distressful daily, continue to adjust your attitude. Thinking positively about diabetes and reframing it helps you create and maintain a good life.

This is an incredibly complex topic. Consider this chapter an aid to your thinking about how you are doing and how you might improve both your self-care and your level of joy. If you know that you are lost in diabetes distress or in depression, seek professional help. Life with type 1 is a tango and your partner will regularly challenge you to learn new steps. Keep dancing.

CHAPTER 8

Sugar in the Blood Goes Up & Down, Up & Down

"Blood sugar for diabetics should be 100," asserted the chiropractor stopping by my table at a health fair. I was offering diabetic education materials and answering questions. I didn't argue with her or try to convince her it wasn't so simple. She was a perfectly distressing example that even alternative health practitioners have fixed ideas about diabetes care and where blood sugar should be. I am thrilled to observe a blood sugar of 100. I go by it often.

My naturopath, who has been a tremendously helpful addition to my health team, thinks any blood glucose over 100 is too high. I don't try to explain to him either. When he asks what my BG (blood glucose) is he gets just one number. He has no idea what journeys my BG and I have undertaken in the hours before meeting with him. Look at the printout of any T1D's blood sugar across time and you will observe significant peaks and valleys.

My point is that blood sugar doesn't stand still. A T1D's blood sugar may take dynamic turns. My blood sugar meanders, speeds up, plunges and then streaks toward the heavens. It regularly transcends borders established by the health care world. And I still manage to stay close to the recommended 7% A1c.

I try to ignore the literature warning that besides high blood sugar these so-called BG excursions cause complications, in particular to my eyes. However carefully I correct my highs and cover carbohydrate intake with insulin, my results will never be as precise as those of a person without diabetes. I am doing my best to act as though I am normal. And I have both an endocrinologist and a diabetes educator to help me.

Despite the intensity of my efforts, my CGM reveals ups and downs, periodically dramatic. There are reasons beyond my daily regimen. There is also *life with diabetes*. Circumstances and bodily fluctuations influence blood sugar. Since insulin is a whimsical hormone that goes its own way, it may behave differently when affected by other hormones. There are several layers of confusing biologic influence. So my pump programming doesn't always match my lifestyle.

Looking at the erratic blood sugar patterns on my CGM report during a visit with my endocrinologist I asked, "What could I do to even out these ups and downs?"

"I have type 1 patients with consistent patterns within the recommended levels," she said. "They eat the same thing every day at the same time. They follow the same routine without much change. I don't see you doing that."

I don't see me doing that either. I exercise on some days and not others. I work on some days and not others. I eat well and cook for myself, restrict carbs and take insulin to cover carbs. But I eat what appeals to me whenever I am hungry. And on occasion I eat badly.

My endocrinologist and others have suggested taking insulin 15 minutes or so before meals or snacks so it can start working as I eat. I have tried that several times and experienced hypoglycemia. Timing is important and so is awareness about what you are eating and when it might raise your blood sugar. Sometimes my food is still cooking and not ready as quickly as I intended. Sometimes my food choices are high fat or otherwise slow to peak. And after many years with diabetes I may have delayed digestion. As an alternative I am investigating inhaled insulin for rapid carb coverage and reducing highs. It is not yet widely used, is expensive, and my insurance doesn't cover it.

Therefore, I work with my patterns constantly. And when a change is clearly needed, I consult with my endocrinologist or diabetes educator and adjust my basal or bolus rates.

Science says...

Research studies involving thousands of people with diabetes have come up with BG numbers that potentially keep us safe from complications. We think the closer to normal BG the better, but there is disagreement about exactly what to aim for.

The American Diabetes Association recommends an average BG of less than 7% (154 mg/dL). The American Association of Clinical Endocrinologists sets 6.5% (140 mg/dL) as the goal. There are further differences for individuals. For example, lower than 8% is thought best for elders or others who might be harmed by hypoglycemia. My own endocrinologist is very happy to observe my A1c at 7.5%. At that average, my CGM shows less than 1% lows, and I am considered safe from serious hypoglycemia.

All the experts currently advise individualizing our self-care, so consider discussing your goals with members of your health care team to find out whether you are in alignment. Your primary care physician, or even your endo, may think your A1c should be different from your own goal. Based on the fact that T2Ds can be very stable and upbeat at 6.5%, many docs think you should be there. However, T1Ds may be utterly wretched at 6.5%, because reaching lower averages might mean we are spending too much time in hypoglycemia.

One diabetes educator told me her whole practice was made up of T1Ds whose quality of life was compromised by going in and out of hypoglycemia trying to stay at 6.5%. Your own experience indicates how harrowing hypoglycemia can be. But now, with CGMs that alert us when we are approaching low blood sugar, many of us are able to live below 7% with minimal hypoglycemia for the first time.

Most type 1s are attempting to stay well, pay attention to recommended BG levels and live happy and healthy lives. Many of those directing us, or just at home loving us, don't realize that our task is close to impossible. Critical and often-unexpected BG ups and downs are part of everyday life for people using exogenous insulin. Even the most mundane tasks may toss us into jeopardy. I might estimate the carbs in my breakfast oatmeal same as yesterday, inject the same amount of insulin as yesterday, and later be either too high or too low. That's not unusual.

Blood sugar is affected by exercise, food, sleep, dehydration, menstruation, menopause, getting the kids off to school, fighting with your spouse and God-knows-what. Highs are certainly harmful, but lows are more immediate and may be more difficult, because when you're low your brain is screaming for fuel and not able to make good judgment calls. Too much of that and your quality of life becomes negligible. Your moods, your energy, your ability to engage and care—all flounder and fluctuate. Is that healthy? Of course not.

Mostly I follow the diabetes *rules*, but I have been called noncompliant by the medical world when doctor's recommendations didn't work for me and I tried to explain. Advice for those with diabetes is often worded as *you should* and *this is what works* and *everyone on insulin has to* and *all type 1s must*. Not only does that assume we are all alike, it talks down to us. Don't you hate being treated like a clueless child? Aren't you supposed to be in charge?

People with diabetes are expected to *control* their diabetes. But of course we can't *control* diabetes. We do our best to *manage* our diabetes, struggling to find balance.

Instead of sinking into the morass of *shoulds* and *oughts*, I recommend you let the outside world dissolve, and turn inward. Consider the possibility of an alliance with your diabetes. Ask yourself:

- How might I learn from, listen to and embrace my diabetes?

- How might I partner with my diabetes to live more gracefully, comfortably, healthily?

- How might this difficult condition aid me?

- How might I be a more complete body/mind/soul with diabetes?

It is one of my deepest beliefs that people with diabetes are integrated resourceful people who happen to have a chronic pay-attention-to-me condition. We are Indy race car drivers and U.S. Supreme Court Justices and NFL champions and rock stars and teachers and nurses and doctors and parents and so much more.

Life with diabetes is complex. Not only do I get angry with the medical world, I get furious at my T1D when it's time to leave for an appointment but first I have to change my insulin pump infusion set and check my blood sugar. I may curse my way through the steps. But then I have to drive to the clinic without road rage, respond nicely to the nurse checking my ascending blood pressure, and answer positively when asked how I am! Hissing and spitting lets off steam, but I try not to stay in that mood long. Anger and resentment don't help me function well. When I am frenetic and bitter, I start to hate myself and I make mistakes. When I lighten up, deep-breathe and admit it's no big deal, I regain my balance. I live in a better place and can take better care of myself.

I am reminded of a disabled war veteran on the news who told his story and how he copes. He said:

1. Stay focused

2. Set small goals

3. Keep going

I do all three. Focusing, setting and accomplishing small goals, I keep going. You can too.

SMBG, A1c & CGM—Blood Sugar Monitoring Advances

High BG is the long-term killer. And low BG is the short-term killer. Balancing between them is the key. How are they measured and how do you know where you stand?

New medications and new technology are emerging at a rapid pace. By the time you read this, technology will have advanced! New types of insulin and drugs to prevent T1D are coming on the market. Some T1Ds are already taking other medications with their insulin, including oral metformin, and injected exenatide (Byetta, Bydureon), liraglutide (Victoza), pramlintide (Symlin), and sitagliptin (Januvia). Plus, the U.S. Food and Drug Administration is investigating sotagliflozin (Zynquista) and TTP399 as adjuncts to insulin.

And medical providers are being urged to evaluate blood sugar control with CGM's glucose management indicator rather than A1cs.

As a backpacker in my twenties, I remember testing urine sugar by peeing onto yellow paper strips that changed color. Even earlier I dropped fat pills into a test tube with a mix of urine and water, where they bubbled into blue for negative and ugly mustard color for high sugar. It took hours for sugar to make it into my urine and there was nothing I could do to address it. But that was all we had at the time.

Sugar in the blood is more immediate than sugar in the urine. Advancements in blood sugar measurement have partnered with improvements in insulin quality and scope. The original insulins made from pork and beef pancreases were replaced by synthetic human insulin and then insulin analogs. They are available in fast-acting, intermediate-acting and long-acting forms. Fast acting forms have developed into rapid-acting, which are not actually rapid. But inhaled insulin acts instantaneously and disappears.

Pricking your finger and feeding a drop of blood onto a strip read by a meter came into usage in the 1980s. It was a miracle! Individuals with diabetes could find out how much sugar was in their blood on their own anywhere anytime. Medical providers have labeled this process SMBG—self-monitoring blood glucose.

Introduction of personal blood sugar meters gave us valuable awareness. I still call them *detective kits* when introducing meters to newly diagnosed people with diabetes. Now when you wonder what your blood sugar is doing you can find out. Meters tell us exactly what our blood sugar is in the moment we check—like a snapshot.

Monitoring was further advanced by introduction of the hemoglobin A1c during the Diabetes Control and Complications Trial, 1983-1993. A1c measures the average amount of glucose bound to hemoglobin in the red blood cells for the past three months. The A1c reveals the central line of blood sugar that averages all your ups and downs over 90 days.

Before the A1c I could be really careful in the hours before a medical appointment and have an excellent BG in my doctor's office. He'd think I was doing fine, congratulate me and send me home without any changes. That could have been the right thing to do, or utterly wrong. All he could see was my BG in that moment. Where had my blood sugar traveled during the months since my last appointment? How high or low had I gone each day? What were my patterns?

Patterns?

Like many T2Ds my dad checked only his fasting blood sugar, which was always near 100. His primary care physician knew a lot about diabetes and checked dad's A1c. It was 9.5% (an average of 226 mg/dL), showing that his blood sugar was going high during the day when he wasn't checking. Grasping the concept of an A1c was difficult. Dad couldn't comprehend why the doctor thought his blood sugar was high when his numbers were perfect every morning.

"Do you ever test after dinner or at bedtime?" I asked. He didn't. I found a diabetes educator near his South Carolina home and urged him to meet with her. They met, and my high school dropout World War II bomber pilot dad was uncharacteristically emotional when he told me later how well she helped him understand the A1c and other concepts that had been difficult for him. With new awareness he accepted his doctor's orders to take a single long-acting insulin shot at bedtime that brought his A1c into the recommended range.

Someone in your family may be confused about the A1c—an average expressed as a percentage. Both average and percentage are terms that may challenge people untrained or uncomfortable with math. Also confusing is that blood sugar meters provide an average. But the meter's blood sugar average is based on the data you enter. My dad had a perfect glucose meter average based on the fasting blood sugars he entered, but he did not test any other time of day. So his meter average was not accurate.

—

Tracking advancements in diabetes care, I want to acknowledge that I have been blessed by technology. Before blood sugar meters became available, and before fast-acting insulin and multiple daily injections, I lived through years of not knowing what my blood sugar was doing or being able to change it. I could only guess whether I was high or low, and couldn't correct highs.

In those times I was living outdoors as much as I could and

intensely physically active. I avoided medical visits and had no diabetes checkups for years. Finally a deep scrape on my shin wouldn't heal and I went to an MD.

At the end of our visit he kindly but firmly advised, "I don't care if you come back to see me. But see a doctor about your diabetes care!"

I did. I saw an endocrinologist and all I remember is that he recommended I start checking my blood sugar with a meter. I said, "No thanks" to the meter suggestion. I still didn't think I needed it. And I had no health insurance to pay for it.

Blurry vision took me to an eye doctor about that time (18 years after diagnosis). My exam revealed diabetic retinopathy, and I immediately underwent my first laser treatment to cauterize those leaky blood vessels. I had to admit that my diabetes wasn't going as well as I had assumed.

My life needed to settle. At 32 years old I stepped from waiting tables and freelance writing to full-time employment. Among my employee benefits was health insurance. That led me to meet with a diabetes educator, accept a blood sugar meter and start multiple daily injections (three or more basal/bolus injections per day). My health and my diabetes awareness improved.

While I was becoming better educated and better managed, technology advanced from finger sticks and meters to measuring diabetes regulation by the hemoglobin A1c. Both are helpful. We can make immediate judgments from single blood sugar results, and also have the A1c's panoramic view. However, for the most part your A1c was checked in your doctor's office or at a lab.

The wheel of fate continued to turn. Diabetes scientists created devices that put blood sugar management back into your own hands. You actually wear the latest advancement—the continuous glucose monitor (CGM). Your CGM communicates through an app on your cell phone or a special monitor. And it might connect with your insulin pump, so you can look at your phone, your monitor or your pump and know your blood sugar number.

You can also allow your doctor or diabetes educator or family and friends to dial into your CGM software program. You and your invited observers can see what your BG average is daily, what time of day you go high or low, and what percentage of time you spend in range. (Time in range is the new standard for people with diabetes, internationally set at 70-180 mg/dL.)

Thanks to CGMs parents of young type 1s can sleep better, receiving alarms when their children's blood sugar is too high or low in the night.

During medical visits both my endocrinologist and my diabetes educator can look at my CGM reports and recommend changes to my carb coverage or basal rate. CGMs are credited with lowering A1c and reducing hypoglycemia. They may also encourage wearers to follow lifestyle recommendations and take medications, because it becomes obvious that they help. Your medical clinic might offer short-term CGMs for you to try. And television commercials for FreeStyle Libre CGMs are currently offering free trials.

But reports indicate that only about 20% of type 1s have CGMs. Not all insurance policies cover them and without insurance coverage they are expensive. I used an insulin pump for almost two years past its 5-year insurance policy until Medicare covered my CGM and I could get approval for the pump it communicated with. Friend Della has a new pump and CGM but they don't communicate. Her insurance company denied coverage for the CGM that talks to her pump because it is more expensive!

The Good, the Bad and the Ugly

Without a CGM, state of the art is to self-monitor blood glucose with strips and a meter. When and how often you check blood glucose depends on your need to know, and advice from your medical provider or diabetes educator. Before my CGM I checked roughly four times a day. When ill or traveling or unusually active I might check up to 10 times a day. Strips are outrageously expensive, so having enough strips is a challenge.

My own insurance no longer covers blood sugar testing strips because the Dexcom G6 CGM I wear supposedly *does not need to be calibrated*. However, 1) you are advised not to treat extreme highs or lows without monitoring first; 2) sometimes the damned CGM transmitter fails and I may have to wait several days until a new one can be delivered; and 3) about one in four times my CGM demands that I calibrate every few hours even though it isn't supposed to. Finally, number 4) it takes two hours for a new sensor to work when I change sites every 10 days, and I may need to check during that time.

As is true in so many instances, the *system* does not respond to real T1D needs. I am buying strips now from a friend whose insurance plan gives him more than enough.

CGM or not, you need a blood sugar meter and strips. How do you know what meter is best? Like everything, it depends. Your diabetes educator probably has information that would help you decide. Clinics, providers and insurance plans usually have favorite

BG meters, or have a financial agreement with a company. Certain meters are thought to be more accurate, but there are standards for meters that must be met, so find one with strips you can afford.

The more you know the better you can choose what works best for your lifestyle. For example, several meters have been manufactured to address disabilities. They talk or can be read by people with low vision. The American Diabetes Association provides information on meters and other gear that makes our lives easier. Click Tools and Support on the ADA home page. Choose Consumer Guide or Devices and Technology.

Money and insurance clearly enter the picture. Whatever the companies manufacturing blood sugar meters claim, the realistic alternative is to find the least expensive BG-testing strips and test as often as you need to. You can live well and stay well using those tools.

Advancements like CGMs, pumps and pens may help but are not necessary. Find your own solutions and know that whatever works for you is the right choice.

Clearly type 1 demands that you make daily and long-term decisions to assure good health. As I grew from teen years into adulthood with T1D, I had my days of upset and resistance. I still have those days. But I know that paying attention to my physical needs serves me. I cannot bury myself in books or my computer and float away. Diabetes reminds me that I live in a body. It grounds me. That is a gift I cannot deny.

- Might your relationship with diabetes have improved your quality of life?

- Does having to pay attention to your diabetes help

you be a better parent, spouse, manager, thinker, artist or citizen?

One diabetes educator told me that diabetes gave her a meaningful career. It has given me a topic that's compelling to write a book about. What has diabetes given you? If you don't know yet, please contemplate how T1D might have helped you become the wise human you are.

Every problem has a gift for you in its hands.

Richard Bach, Author of 25 Books including *Jonathan Livingston Seagull*

CHAPTER 9

Tango Instead of Fight

Relentlessly the headlines, the websites and the public service announcements insist that we attack, subdue, eliminate, destroy diabetes. I listened to a PBS special today and once again I am urged to join the *War on Diabetes*.

But I am not a killer and I refuse to live at war. When my blood sugar won't settle down and my eyes are blurry and my skin itches and I have no energy, I cannot rally and fight. Who would I be fighting? I have type 1 diabetes so I would be fighting myself.

Instead I employ empathy and connection. I comfort myself. I imagine celebrating peace with diabetes and stepping into a dance. I use words like embrace, unite with, learn from and validate. I seek a true alliance—creating opportunities to know and value and perhaps even (on my good days) love my diabetes. I choose the image of myself artistically advancing across a dance floor with my partner, immersed in mutual movement. I visualize myself at one with my diabetes.

Of all the forms of dance on earth, I chose the tango as my metaphor for dancing with diabetes. I have not danced an actual tango and only know what I read and watch—the statuesque and compelling interaction of partners dancing closely. I can imagine myself following the steps of this elaborate dance, greatly moved and not sure whether to laugh at myself or cry at the beauty of the dance.

Why the tango?

At the heart of tango (Argentine tango) is the desire to listen to, understand and converse with the person you're dancing with, through this unique language of dance. So, tango can be many things for different people.

http://www.tangolingua.com/what-is-tango

Traditional tango enthusiasts recognize the depth of expression that is possible through the tango. Dancing with my own type 1 diabetes might be vibrant and playful one day and heartbreaking the next. Tango partners alternate as leaders and followers. As I continue to tango with type 1 diabetes, I discover more about myself as well as my consort.

Tango triumphs for a unique reason. While most dances are created to celebrate life, tango serves a different purpose. It is created by the least fortunate to shelter their sorrows. They do not come to the milonga to play peacocks, but to expose their vulnerability and seek comfort, to dance the loneliness, homesickness, nostalgia, and grief in them, to find a shoulder to rely on, to take refuge for their wounds, to quench their thirst for love, and to touch and be touched by another human being....

https://yangningyuan.blogspot.com/2012/03/
why-people-dance-tango.html

My heart is full as I read these definitions. They refer to the whole range of living, from vibrant and playful to vulnerable and grieving. In my tango with diabetes I seek comfort while dancing the difficulty of living with a sometimes-limiting partner. Even with the latest technological backup, those of us linked with type 1 stand at every moment close to death. But with a deeply curious attitude, our humanity is intensified. More emotions and a wider range of living are available to all of us with T1D.

—

What type 1 diabetes has taught me is very personal and what it will teach you is also unique. Even when intimately associated with a sweetheart or a dear friend, I struggle to explain all that T1D encompasses. My life work has been to learn more about myself, to express my soul's truth in my daily life, to live inside my complex body. Diabetes aids me in that quest. I allow greater awareness as I embrace this partnership.

In a certain sense, diabetes is wrapped around and through my whole life. When I am on a car trip, I have plotted out where to stop to check all my diabetes gear and reports, and what to have within reach for low blood sugar. I have food for several days because I never know what I will find when I'm away from home. My phone is face up on the seat beside me so I can hear it beep blood sugar alarms.

I imagine myself to be like the attentive parent of a small child. I need to stay in full awareness at all times and to have appropriate accoutrements for all eventualities! Of course, that's impossible, but it's my aim. I worry as I fall asleep whether my blood sugar will go dangerously up or down while I am slumbering. When I am at a party or driving home from one, I wonder whether the alcohol I drank will send me too low, and how I could convince a police officer that I am not drunk if I am stopped with low blood sugar. I doubt I could walk a straight line. God knows I've imagined being jailed by police who won't let me take my insulin. Every challenging episode, real and imagined, reminds me of my sensitivity, which I transform into a remarkable and valuable trait. I tell myself how fortunate I am to be so in tune with my physical self.

But there are always surprises, and there is always a need for close attention. Driving to work on the interstate one morning my hands began shaking. Trees and shrubs along the highway were not moving so I knew there was no wind. I pulled off at the next exit and checked my blood sugar: 50 mg/dL. I went inside the convenience store and bought juice. Drank the juice, waited 15 minutes and checked again. Still 50. I bought and drank more juice. Fifteen minutes later my glucose was 80. I pulled back onto the highway.

I could be angry at my diabetes. I could be angry at myself. But I prefer visualizing myself engaged in a tango, expressing my upset creatively as I drink juice and count minutes. Driving on toward work I smile, and when I reach my office and leave my car, I bow to my invisible partner and walk inside. I stamp my timecard, and my supervisor greets me. "You're late. Can't have that. Make it by 8 a.m. or you will be written up."

"Yes," I answer. She is not a supporter of mine and considers any physical episode my diabetes might cause a lapse in judgment, so it is useless to explain. Also, useless to blame myself or to step into the inner darkness of being misunderstood. Best to think of that episode as another tango. My T1D partner arrived unexpectedly and demanded that we dance. I responded appropriately.

Having type 1 diabetes keeps me in close touch with myself and has shaped me. If a cure comes in my lifetime, I will receive it gratefully. But meanwhile I choose to embrace diabetes as an asset to my existence.

Certainly my existence with diabetes has not always been a tango. However, in my lifelong journey I have become more adept at choosing how I respond and what I create. My emotional reactions to the demands and disturbances associated with my diabetes have shifted over the years. And, of course, I still have full-on cursing and kicking moments.

All my emotions are real and valuable. They may be triggered by the meanderings of blood sugar but am I able to channel my emotions in a way that serves me? I believe I have choices. I am not at the mercy of whatever happens to me. I always have choice.

Country music singer and talk show host Kelly Clarkson ends every show saying, "Have a great day and if it's not great, change it." I love her for that. When my day gets rocky and T1D is demanding, I can change it.

No one knows exactly how our emotions come about. Psychologists and philosophers associate emotions with thoughts, physical sensations and our personal and cultural backgrounds. Part of expressing my true self and applying creativity may be to track and to reconsider my emotional responses.

An example I hear about from many sources is reinterpreting fear as anticipation. Maybe you are meeting your fiancée's family for the first time, starting a new job, or anticipating lab results. When you think about it your breath quickens, your throat squeezes a little, and the skin on your arms shivers. You can name those responses fear or anticipation. Both are potentially true. For a happier life I choose to call my responses anticipation.

Everything is energy and energy ebbs and flows. Consider where you are in your diabetes journey. What makes you happy, worried, sad or angry? Use your splendid imagination to enhance your positive feelings and let the negative ones be felt, acknowledged, and then drift away. Use the tools you have developed in your lifetime of learning.

One way I change my mood is to leave whatever I'm doing for a while and take a walk. I put my phone in my pocket so I can easily grab it and record random thoughts. I breathe, listen, look, open and close my hands, wiggle my toes as I walk. Movement engages me. Neighborhood birds carry on volubly while devouring seeds and fruits in the cedars and pyracantha. My mind shifts into happier and more creative modes.

Physical freedom and being in nature are strong values of mine. I am so grateful to have mobility. Years ago, I drew a circle around my location on the state map—measuring how many miles I could comfortably drive round trip in a day. Within that circle I have explored and found places of great natural beauty and peacefulness that help me return to my true self.

In times and places where I cannot go to a special location or be in nature—like inside a major airport—I center my sight on a tree or a patch of grass or the cloudy sky beyond the window. Or I have a pebble in my pocket that I can hold tightly while I breathe and remember where I picked it up.

We are living on earth, and being rooted here is valuable. When I was an Outward Bound instructor, I demonstrated the value of grounding before we hiked along a narrow path with exposure to the cliffs below. I had my students place their feet firmly on the ground and imagine sending roots down into the earth. We tried lifting one another before and after that exercise and students were always amazed when they got heavier after envisioning rootedness.

I hope that all of you reading this can stand and walk. If you cannot, let whatever part of your body is nearest the ground send down those roots, and move however you can. From that in-your-body rooted-in-the-earth place, come back to yourself. Make your own music with your thoughts and even your heartbeats. Imagine stepping into a tango with your diabetes. Practice makes perfect. You can get used to the idea of dancing rather than fighting or denying or raging against your diabetes and its challenges. You can settle into a tough situation with a smile, knowing that you are becoming expert at dancing with a very difficult partner in a very difficult dance.

Although when danced by professionals the tango looks intricate, it's actually based on walking, and is therefore considered a dance for everyone. Whoever we are and whatever we know, we can invent a personal tango with T1D. Since our dance is entirely in our imagination we can quickly excel. We will be better at it some days than others and able to dance with some issues better than others. But instead of fighting we can dance. I stamp my feet and whirl into my tango, grateful for all that I have, all that I know, all that I am. And I respond to my diabetes partner's dips and turns, ever more sure of myself.

PART 4

LIFESTYLE CHANGE

CHAPTER 10

You Can't Eat That!

Unhelpful advice about what I should eat is rampant, and still angers me after all my years with diabetes. Walking into a massage school for a demonstration of foot reflexology, I was greeted by the school director. She welcomed me, invited me to help myself to refreshments, and asked why I had come.

"I have diabetes and I work with people who have diabetes, so I am interested in how reflexology might help," I replied.

She picked up the tray of cookies on the refreshment table and whirled it away, saying, "You can't eat this."

I didn't slap her. I couldn't even look at her. And I didn't reply. I hadn't planned to eat one of her damned cookies anyway. But she was the leader of a training program for healers. I had given a talk to one of her classes about diabetes. She should have known better. I turned around and moved into the classroom, where I sat in the front row with smoke rising out of my ears.

Most type 1s are planning every minute what we must do and must not do. Being told "You can't eat that!" by a stranger who has no idea what I can or can't eat is maddening. I have had type 1 diabetes for more than 60 years! The very fact that I'm alive makes me an expert.

As a graduate student in a University of New Mexico Public Health class I experienced another of those exasperating events. Filling my plate at a potluck during a break from class I took an oatmeal cookie. The woman behind me sputtered, "You can't eat that." I glared at her, left my food and slammed out of the room. After circling the building four times, cursing and breathing hard, I came back and took the professor aside.

"May I act out an issue with diabetes for our class?" I asked.

She agreed and reconvened the students. I pretended to check my blood sugar and look at the foods offered. I talked to myself as I filled an imaginary plate.

"My blood sugar is perfect and I'm hungry. I can have a flour tortilla with beans and cheese and salsa. One apple would be all right. I'll inject insulin to cover the carbs I'm eating. And the cookies look so good! I can check my blood sugar again after class and eat the cookie on my long drive home."

Turning to my audience I said, "I am thinking all the time about what will work for me and what I need to do. When someone is sure they know better than I do and says, 'You can't eat that,' I want to scream and smack them!"

Several of the students listening were crying. Their chorus was, "I want to help my friend with diabetes (or spouse or brother or parent) but I don't know what to do."

I advised, "In a peaceful moment when it's not mealtime, tell them you love them and want to know how to help. Assume nothing."

What people with type 1 diabetes can or cannot eat is always an issue, and apparently every human being on the planet has an opinion, many documented in *New York Times* best sellers. Even though certain recommendations are considered good for all, everyone deals with foods differently. Each of us will find foods that work well and others that upset our nutritional balance or send our blood sugar higher than expected.

Many health professionals believe that all sugar should be banned for those with diabetes, even natural sugars. Other experts believe type 1s can eat anything they want to eat!

We *can* eat anything. But eating indiscriminately is dangerous. We do need to attend to our choosy bodies. Regularly consuming foods that lack true nourishment or need massive insulin doses weakens us. For ongoing health, type 1s need foods that nurture us, keep our blood sugar in our target range, and don't upset our health balance. How will you know if what you eat contributes to your health? Certain foods are obviously not for everyday consumption. Life experience and individualized expert advice will help us sort out the rest.

Early Warning

I must confess that despite plenty of life experience, there are times I don't listen to what I know. I adopt one of my former husband's smart-ass sayings, "If you're gonna do it, you might as well overdo it!"

Months into the pandemic with an election brewing and Covid-19 cases rising, I definitely overdid it! I added pasta to both lunch and dinner several times a week. I picked up treats from a restaurant that served exquisite carrot cake. And I discovered gluten free ice cream cones. I hadn't eaten an ice cream cone in years so I bought three boxes of cones and three pints of ice cream. Without a second thought, I began eating ice cream cones every day.

Over those weeks of eating foolishly, my macular edema worsened and I woke each morning with blurry vision. I was exhausted, discouraged and not sleeping well. It didn't occur to me that the comfort food I was overdoing was disturbing my body's equilibrium.

With my endocrinologist's advice I altered my insulin basal rate to address *unexplained* high blood sugar. I had not yet made the connection between my pasta/cake/ice cream binge and troubles, so I didn't reveal my questionable food choices.

Then I recounted the physical changes that were scaring me to my chiropractor/naturopath Tom, who has significant training in nutrition. I knew he would criticize my carb extravagance, so I didn't tell him what I had been eating either. He listened to me and checked my pulses.

"Your body is showing a high rate of inflammation and trying to process more sugar than it can handle," Tom concluded. He recommended avoiding all carbohydrates except vegetables and fruit for two weeks. Although ordinarily I ignore his ultra-low-carb recommendations, this time I agreed with him. I cut out the treats and went keto.

That experience revealed that although my best resource may be experience, occasionally I lose my mind. Turning to my health team helps me get back to smart thinking. I stop criticizing myself and acknowledge that diabetes does create limits. Thinking positively, I assume that my type 1 alarm system supports me by demanding that I eat well and pay attention.

You may already have figured this out. And you may have discovered foods that don't work. You may even—like me—have eaten them anyway. Hopefully you have a recovery plan for getting quickly back on track. It is vital to know that you can go astray and come back.

A recovery plan may even be necessary when we eat well, because our bodies constantly respond to change, good or bad. Nutrition needs fluctuate with positive events like a vacation, wedding, graduation, pregnancy, promotion or retirement. And our bodies change with the more often recognized challenges of job loss, injury, grief or a life-threatening diagnosis. During those times we might support ourselves by being stricter with our nutrition rather than grasping questionable food for comfort. Or we might have to find a new way entirely.

Essential tactics for establishing and maintaining your best eating plan include flexibility and continuing to educate yourself, because recommendations keep changing and we keep changing. You may find out more about what to eat and drink by working with a savvy dietitian or an alternative practitioner. And taking loved ones to your appointment might be helpful for support in your personal relationships as well as for their better understanding.

Here are a few basics to keep in mind:
- Type 1s need to nurture our bodies overall, as does everyone.

- Carbohydrates are the foods that raise blood sugar. We need a certain number of carbohydrates for energy and for our brains to think clearly. Too many carbs will send us right over the cliff—like Wily Coyote endlessly chasing the Roadrunner.

- Part of the challenge and satisfaction of taking care of yourself with diabetes is establishing your own eating plan. It is neither simple nor easy. Finding your way demands clarity of body, mind and perhaps heart. Some obstacles will be discussed as you read on.

- Overall, the many sides of you that get involved with food may cause confusion. Experiencing pain or fear or rebellion, for example, may alter your true perception. And, like me, you may not always listen to your wiser self.

- Type 1s MUST count carbs. Knowing what will raise your blood sugar, and how much, starts with counting the carbohydrates you plan to consume. Counting carbs and knowing how to cover them with insulin is the gold standard for keeping blood sugar in range. I turn to my diabetes educator and endocrinologist for help with that.

- Expert advice can help, but be careful who you listen to. Find a smart and kind diabetes educator or dietitian familiar with type 1s. Make sure they know you—your culture, your habits, your financial limits, your social life, your levels of stress and exercise, and what you crave! Weigh the possibilities. Consider alternatives.

- And always know that you keep changing.

—

The American Diabetes Association (ADA) looked into this topic in July 2019 and concluded that there is no *diabetes diet* that's good for everyone. Briefly, the ADA concluded:

> Everyone's body responds differently to different types of foods and diets, so there is no single "magic" diet for Diabetes.

Since everyone's body responds differently to foods we eat, we need to find our own dietary plans and keep learning. Remember that everyone has an opinion, but you know the most about your body. I overheard a long conversation between a client and the dietitian who works with me. The client had received so much advice on what she should eat that she had no idea what to do. The dietitian's advice was, "Don't listen to anyone else. Choose something and start."

Where to start?

WARNING

I am NOT a dietitian. I counsel my clients on general nutrition for diabetes management and refer them to a registered dietitian for Medical Nutrition Therapy. What I include here is easily available information from sources including the American Diabetes Association and American Heart Association, with tips from my own experience.

My first advice is to stop sugared beverages, including fruit juice. An apple may be an excellent snack for you. But a glass of apple juice is missing the natural roughage (fiber) that helps your body use the apple in the best possible way. And how many apples were juiced to fill the glassful you drank at lunch?

Second, select foods as close as possible to how they grow. Foods that are less processed, less changed or interfered with, will sustain you. How far has that cornflake or corn chip come from a kernel on the corncob growing in your garden? What was stripped away that could have nurtured your body and kept your blood sugar steady?

Third, I solidly back the American Heart Association's emphasis on quality. Grow your own or buy the freshest food you can find and the best you can afford.

Fourth, experiment to determine your own nutritional plan. Diabetes has helped me find a way of eating that nurtures me and is very satisfying. Rather than feeling limited, I call myself a picky eater. My example of overdoing indicates that I am not a saint. But being a picky eater works for me 99% of the time. For the most part, I choose high quality delicious food, eat lots of vegetables, and restrict carbohydrates. I prepare my own snacks and meals. Except for potato chips—my downfall—I am not drawn to junk food. And when we are celebrating birthdays at work, I know the cake came from the grocery store. It's too sweet and made from cheap ingredients. I don't want even a bite.

What guidelines will you establish? How will you get to a healthier place when you love to eat what you know isn't good for you? I started out by buying or making a treat as similar to the *not-so-good* choice as I could. For example, when I visited my mother in South

Carolina we went to a strawberry farm and picked bucketsful of berries. In the kitchen later, mother sugared a cupful of the berries, piled them on angel food cake and slathered it all with sweetened whipped topping. She ate that concoction while I made my own fake strawberry shortcake. I sliced strawberries onto a whole grain piece of toast, topped it with thick plain yogurt, cinnamon and a drizzle of maple syrup. Delicious!

Your taste buds will change as you proceed with your better and better food plan. Overly sweet or salty foods and many fast foods lack subtle flavoring, and we usually gobble our burgers and fries instead of savoring every bite. As you adjust what you eat to better sustain your health, you will also open the door to more delicious and satisfying foods. Soon just-picked berries or a fresh asparagus spear or an apple right off the tree will stop you in your tracks with flavor, color and texture. Food becomes an adventure and a treasure.

Consider new discoveries. Try raw oysters, truffles, odiferous cheeses, dim sum and falafel. When you're cooking at home add herbs and spices and ingredients you haven't tasted before. Experiment with unknown vegetables. Or try a new way to prepare something familiar. For example, with an inexpensive spiralizer you can turn zucchini into long strands like spaghetti. Dress it with pesto or tomato sauce and avoid the carbs in traditional pasta.

Part of your food adventure will be finding out how a new choice treats your body. Evaluate your blood sugar before and two hours after you eat to find out how well it works for you.

If you cannot even imagine eating like this, or food doesn't seem that important, give yourself a hug for even reading about it. There's a wonderful little boy in a highchair that I've seen several times on

TV. He has given me a phrase I use when I don't want to do what I think I should. That baby's mother asks if he wants a serving of vegetables. He smiles and sings, "Not today."

Maybe not today but soon, you might begin by eating whatever you eat with greater awareness. Stop to eat, savor what you eat. Let food be more important rather than less. Begin to build in goodness step-by-step. Remember that you want to live long and well. Be curious about how you might adapt your eating habits to help you do that. Make changes when you are ready.

Once you decide to give eating well a priority, keep reading.

Be skeptical, ask questions, demand proof. Demand evidence. Don't take anything for granted. But here's the thing: When you get proof, you need to accept the proof. And we're not that good at doing that.

Michael Specter
American Journalist and Author of *Denialism*

CHAPTER 11

What Can You Eat?

Wherever you live there are wonderful foods that will keep you healthy and happy. However, essential to any eating plan—carbohydrates raise blood sugar. Let yourself recognize carbs and have a healthy respect for them. Two important learning curves will make a difference for you: knowing your food groups and counting your carbohydrates.

I simplify those choices for my clients with a food group handout I co-created with a dietitian, and a second one that shows carb portion sizes. (You can find both pages on my website.) The food group handout lists and has pictures of proteins, non-starchy vegetables, fats and carbohydrates. The carbs include sweets, fruits, dairy products, grains, starchy vegetables and junk food.

The portion page has been a tremendous aid for me and my clients and started excellent conversations. Consider creating a page that lists portions for your favorite carbohydrates.

Practice by evaluating the carbs in your breakfast.

- Half a cup of cooked oatmeal is one portion (15 grams) of carbohydrate. I bet your oatmeal serving measures more than half a cup.

- Is it instant or do you cook it?

- What do you put on your oatmeal?
    > A serving of one cup of oatmeal with half a cup of milk, a handful of raisins and half a banana adds up to 4 or 5 portions of carbohydrate.

    > You might add a piece of toast—at least one more portion of carbs.

    > Or...

When I taught my nondiabetic but always eager to lose weight mother about carbs, she changed her breakfast routine. (Many of us believe that overabundance of carbohydrates causes weight gain.) She reduced carbs by putting fresh blueberries in her oatmeal instead of raisins and a banana, eating just one piece of toast and adding an egg. Protein is a good partner for carbohydrates. It doesn't raise blood sugar, adds a feeling of satiety and helps your meal stick with you longer.

Learning to count carbs effectively and pare them down with satisfying alternatives makes good after-meal blood sugar possible.

There are a number of ways to get even more careful with your choices. One is to most often choose what are called complex carbo-hydrates. Complex carbs are absorbed more slowly than simple carbs so may be less likely to spike your blood sugar. Complex carbs include whole oats, brown rice, quinoa, beans and lentils.

Some simple carbohydrates are white bread, white rice, mashed potatoes, sugar, milk and all fruits. If your breakfast choices are all simple carbs, that might send your blood sugar high for the whole day. But *your* body may not care whether your carb choices are simple or complex. Find out for yourself.

As you try different combinations or ways to prepare them, you will become ever more aware of how your choices work. Whole grains are better for all of us. But they do raise blood sugar. And even though fruits are simple carbohydrates, most fresh fruits contain fiber, which slows down their absorption. Some high-fiber fruits are berries, kiwis, cherries, pomegranates, pears and oranges. Dried fruits are high in fiber too but concentrated so very sweet. Fresh fruit is a better choice for keeping your blood sugar in a good place.

Type 1s sometimes calculate *net carbs* by subtracting fiber from a food's carb count, because fiber is all or partially undigested. Keto diet enthusiasts work with net carbs. And manufacturers emphasize net carbs to sell their products. However, calculating net carbs is controversial and not scientifically backed. The American Diabetes Association does not use the term net carbs. They recommend always looking at total carbohydrates on the nutrition facts label and checking your blood sugar to be sure how specific carbs affect you.

The *glycemic index* is another term some nutrition enthusiasts use. The Academy of Nutrition & Dietetics explains, "The glycemic index, simply put, is a measure of how quickly a food causes our blood sugar levels to rise."

A Harvard Medical School article in January 2020 explained

that a low score on the glycemic index indicates foods that release glucose slowly and steadily (barley, rolled oats, apples, kidney beans, soy milk). Foods higher on the index release glucose more rapidly (bread, instant oats, watermelon, mashed potatoes, rice milk).

I don't subtract fiber from my carb counts and I don't consciously use the glycemic index. It makes sense that brown rice is better for me than white and rolled oat flakes have more nutritional value than packets of chopped up instant oats. The overall food awareness I have developed over time, and knowing or looking up the carb count for my food choices, helps me stay healthy. As you pay closer attention and learn more you will match your food awareness skills with your lifestyle to keep your body purring along.

The American Diabetes Association offers further advice.

- Eating doesn't have to be boring.

- It's all about finding the right balance that works for you.

- Regardless of what cuisine you prefer, all healthy eating plans include:
    > Fruits and vegetables
    > Lean meats and plant-based sources of protein
    > Less added sugar
    > Less processed foods

That's good advice. However, one change I sincerely wish the ADA and everyone advising us about food would make is to list *vegetables and fruits* instead of *fruits and vegetables*. Emphasize vegetables! Put them first. That simple change could make a big difference in how people in the U.S. think about healthy eating.

Types of Diets

Many of my clients, my friends, professional athletes, movie stars, television commentators and people interviewed on the street are looking for structured eating plans that feed them well and simplify their lives. Whatever health reasons motivate us, we look for food guidelines.

"Give me a list of what to eat," one of my clients insisted. I can suggest, because selecting a particular diet or following menus may provide helpful structure, especially as he begins his type 1 food journey. But he has to find his own way through the nutrition jungle.

Whether you have diabetes or not, a new diet may be life changing. I follow championship tennis and I read years ago that Serbian Novak Djokovic was collapsing during matches. His legs stopped working, he fell, he vomited, he couldn't breathe. With help from a nutritionist he discovered that foods he depended on were harming his body. He made a number of difficult dietary changes that built his strength and ushered him into a series of tennis championships. In 2013 Djokovic explained his changes in his book, *Serve to Win: The 14-Day Gluten-Free Plan for Physical and Mental Excellence.* (Note the inclusion of mental excellence in his title.)

Djokovic discovered that he was allergic to both wheat and dairy products. His diet now is based on vegetables, beans, fruit, nuts, seeds, lentils, healthy oils and occasional fish. His menus incorporate the ideals of several official diets. And he has made mealtime a healthy ritual, starting with prayer and concentrating on his food as he eats.

Former tennis champion and commentator John McEnroe laughed at his own past when commenting on Djokovic's changes. McEnroe said he and co-champ Jimmy Connors played professional tennis in the 1980s when monetary prizes were slim. To compete at Wimbledon, they scraped together the air fare, and once in London subsisted on the cheapest fish and chips they could find! Looking at photos of skinny McEnroe in his prime, and muscular Djokovic, points out changes in societal health awareness. We are cognizant now that athletes depend on their bodies and those bodies need to be well fed. And type 1s depend on our bodies and our bodies need to be well fed.

You may be aided by a specific meal plan developed with the help of a registered dietitian, especially if you are sensitive to certain foods. Meanwhile, there are a few diets you might investigate that are widely used and backed by experts.

The **Mediterranean-style** diet is based on the traditional foods of people living around the Mediterranean Sea. My parents lived near the Mediterranean in Turkey for two years when I was in my mid-twenties and I spent several weeks with them. In the morning my mother hired a donkey cart and was trotted to the local market to buy the day's vegetables and fruits. She loved to cook and gave recipes and advice to other American women who didn't know what to do with fresh food! Breakfast in a Turkish restaurant was a treat I have long remembered. We were served small glasses of hot and strong black tea, crusty sourdough bread, olives and, by request for an American, a soft-boiled egg.

Numerous countries, cultures, religions and ethnicities are represented near the Mediterranean. Despite their differences, most share these qualities in their cuisine:

- an abundance of fresh vegetables, fruits, herbs and spices, grown nearby
- whole grains, potatoes, beans, nuts and seeds, also grown nearby
- olive oil
- fish and poultry rather than red meat
- fewer dairy products, eggs and meat than we eat in the U.S.
- low to moderate servings of wine, usually with meals
- limited sweets, more often fruit for dessert
- no sugar-sweetened, processed or refined foods or beverages

The American Heart Association recommends a Mediterranean-style diet and also endorses **DASH** (Dietary Approaches to Stop Hypertension). DASH includes more dairy products and meat than a Mediterranean-style diet and does not depend on olive oil. The Heart Association also admits that vegetarian or vegan diets may be good choices.

A third-generation Italian friend of mine was already eating an excellent primarily vegetarian diet when she discovered that her cholesterol was high. Helen refused to take medication to reduce her cholesterol. Instead, she conducted deep research and created a food plan she loves that brought her cholesterol into the recommended range. There's no meat or sugar in her diet and whole grains are cooked into soups and stews rather than ground into flour. Her amazing salads mix ingredients like broccoli, kale and cauliflower, quinoa, red onion, sunflower seeds, jicama, lentils or beans. She's a gardener and a cook so this is a natural lifestyle for her. Though I like sharing what she prepares, I am not willing to change my food routine quite that much. My balance is to eat well *and* take cholesterol-lowering medication. There's always choice.

Consider the assets and liabilities of further dietary styles. The **keto(genic)** diet, generally consisting of 5% carbs, 15% protein and 80% fat, is quite controversial but has strong supporters. My beautiful artist neighbor in her forties eats avocados, meat, fish and eggs. Her favorite snack is chicharrons (fried pork rinds). Olivia also needs a fiber laxative to help her body move out her food choices. She enjoys the way she eats and stays slim and active. But nutrition experts wonder about long-term effects of the keto diet. (Some people say they were diagnosed with type 1 and got off insulin because they are following a keto diet. I have not looked into that so don't know. It is my understanding that we type 1s need at least basal insulin forever.)

Occasional **fasting** is considered a positive health choice by some nutritional advisers. Although it's possible, extended fasting is not generally recommended for people with type 1 diabetes. I have fasted only briefly when directed to by my doctor prior to surgery or a colonoscopy, and in that case, I had clear juice on hand in case of hypoglycemia.

However, intermittent fasting offers several ways to limit eating, and is a choice particularly appealing for those seeking weight loss. Some proponents recommend *alternate day fasting*, when you eat normally one day and limit calories or carbs the following day. The doctor and nurses I worked with in a small rural clinic practiced the 5:2 plan. They ate a regular healthy diet 5 days a week and cut down to 500-800 calories on the other 2 days. They found the 5:2 plan achievable, and appreciated the results, claiming it gave them energy as well as initiating moderate weight loss. They scheduled their fasting days for work time. So they had ample support, and their low-calorie eating didn't interfere with family life.

The 5:2 plan uses calories to limit foods, but carbohydrates can be substituted. Thebloodsugardiet.com addresses this:

> We recommend that you follow a relatively low carbo-hydrate Mediterranean style diet on your fasting days which incorporates plenty of protein (as this cannot be stored) such as fish/seafood, chicken, eggs, beans, tofu, seeds, legumes and nuts.

Time-restricted eating is another fasting approach. You select an 8-hour eating period, say 10 a.m. to 6 p.m., and then fast until 10 a.m. the following day. Type 1s could certainly choose that approach, possibly adjusting their basal insulin to keep their blood sugar from going too low.

And many diabetes educators and dietitians use one of several **plate methods** to teach people with diabetes how to eat. Plate images are colorful and easy to follow, with realistic artwork or photos of good foods. Those methods use a 9-inch plate, which is smaller than most dinner plates. About half the plate is meant to be filled with vegetables. One fourth is meant to contain protein. And the remaining one-fourth of the plate serves for carbohydrates, with fruit or a sweet beverage like milk on the side.

These are only a few of myriad possibilities. Read about whatever diet intrigues you. Combine the most compelling aspects of several diet plans. Or follow a particular one if that will streamline and improve your nutritional approach. Discuss individualizing any plan with a dietitian. Perhaps add the perspective of an alternative nutrition specialist. Blood tests or hair analysis can specify allergies or nutritional needs. Your plan will expand and improve over time as you discover what fosters your nutritional health and satisfaction.

Like Djokovic you may discover food sensitivities that call for medical advice and further restructuring of your food plan. Don't worry. The world is full of delectable healthy food. You may just have to search a little harder.

Eating for celiac disease or gluten intolerance is an additional complication. See a dietitian, read studies and reports and use the same principles that are covered here. One warning—many gluten-free choices are higher in carbs than wheat. For example, rice flour is often the primary ingredient in gluten-free breads and pasta. And rice is high carb. One very thin slice of a local gluten free bread I eat has 26 grams of carbohydrate. Instead, most whole-grain store-bought breads with gluten are about 15 grams of carbohydrate per slice. Check the label on the bag your bread comes in or ask the baker for a carb count so you can cover it properly with your insulin dose.

Eating Out

When planning a restaurant visit, consider your options ahead of time. Read the menu online and choose your meal before you go. Call the chef if you want details. To manage carbs, you might eat half of a large entrée and bring the rest home for later. You might request a special entree made just for you. Or you could tell your waiter to skip the side of rice and add more vegetables.

For more ideas, read on.

*The fridge had been emptied of all Dudley's favorite things —
fizzy drinks and cakes, chocolate bars and burgers — and filled
instead with fruit and vegetables and the sorts of things that
Uncle Vernon called "rabbit food."*

J.K. Rowling
Author of Harry Potter Books

CHAPTER 12

Lesser-Known Food Facts
Fats, Flavor, Labels, Counting Carbs, Sugar-Free Foods & Sugar Substitutes

The famous Southern chef Paula Deen, who promoted sweet desserts and fatty fried foods in her cookbooks and restaurants, was diagnosed with type 2 diabetes in 2008. She was terribly shocked, disappeared from the public eye for months, and recreated her recipes to make them diabetes-friendly. For herself, she came up with a Sunday plan. She eats well all week but allows herself to eat anything she wants on Sundays. That plan has succeeded for her. She lost weight and leveled her blood sugar. A Sunday plan for you as a type 1 could be more complicated. But be creative. How can you maintain your love of food, enjoy eating and spare the carbs and bad fats?

Finding your food path is an all-encompassing process. We naturally have attachments to certain foods. Changing our ways is hard. Economics channel our choices. Emotions may determine both what food or drink we yearn for and what we actually purchase. In some cultures, it is risky to stand out, so eating differently may draw criticism or set us apart.

Where you live has an impact on what you eat. Both city and rural folks may live in what are called *food deserts*. That means their choices are limited by what is sold nearby. And what is sold nearby may not be healthy.

Holidays you were raised with might be linked with certain foods and beverages you know no longer work for you. Acknowledge that some foods need to be left behind. And certain foods feed your heart, so you will find a way to include but limit them. Don't criticize yourself if you briefly step into bad habits. Hug yourself and start over.

Some Thoughts

- Another description for carbohydrates is comfort food.

- Limiting carbohydrates may feel like self-denial.

- Cultures and families impact what we consider good food.

- Income affects what we are able to buy.

    > Food insecurity complicates. When a family has not eaten for three days and a paycheck arrives, doughnuts may be first choice.

    > Inequalities in our world have forced many people to get their food from food banks. They are not able to pick and choose. If that is true for you or someone you know please accept my compassion. Do your best with what you are given. Stay active to burn off extra carbs.

Good Fats/Bad Fats

Nutrition specialists no longer advise us to eat low-fat or no-fat. We are instead invited to concentrate on good fats.

- Avocados, nuts, olive oil and canola oil are examples of good fats.

- Everyone needs good fats.

- Animal fats, like lard and bacon, are not so good—harder for our bodies to use well.

- Nutritionists used to tell people to eat margarine instead of butter. Now they say don't eat margarine, and you can eat a little butter. European chefs often cook with olive oil and add just a touch of butter for flavor.

- Trans fats (trans fatty acids) are made in an industrial process that adds hydrogen to liquid vegetable oils to make them more solid. Also known as partially hydrogenated oils, they are *not* considered safe in human food. They are still broadly used, but a warning must be posted on food packaging. Avoid them.

- Good fats eaten with carbohydrates slow absorption and help keep blood sugar from spiking. The fat in dark chocolate or cheesecake, for example, makes them good choices for type 1s who want to enjoy a sweet.

- And fats eaten when a person with diabetes has low

blood sugar are a bad choice because they will slow your rise to normal. I learned that the hard way when I got very low near an ice cream shop and ate a scoop. The high-fat ice cream stopped my blood sugar from rising so I had to drink juice too and wait longer than usual to recover.

Flavor

Working for a caterer as a party boss, I picked up food and supplies and proceeded to homes or social venues to serve special-occasion meals. When people complimented his foods, the caterer smiled and thanked them. Then he whispered to me, "Sugar, salt and fat." Those are the components of flavor and that's very helpful information. For example, know that when a chef or manufacturer takes out one of those flavor enhancers, the other two might be increased. Low-fat foods may be extra salty or sweet. Low-salt foods may have more fat. And so on.

That leads to a downside of low-fat, no-fat foods for people with type 1 diabetes. How do they affect your blood sugar? Fat usually helps. Milk, for example, is sweet, no matter whether you choose whole milk, 2%, 1% or no fat. But whole milk may suit type 1s better because the natural fat included slows down the absorption of sugar.

Also helpful to know is that as we age many of us lose taste sensation. For that reason, we may add extra salt, fat or sweetness so our foods still taste good. My type 2 dad showered his meals with salt even before tasting. And he frequented a restaurant during senior half-price hours where he could splurge at the dessert bar. I was less judgmental when I learned that age had reduced his capacity to taste his food. I spoke with his doctor and helped arrange insulin coverage for his sweet tooth extravagances.

What to Read on Labels

In the U.S., packaged foods must have nutritional labels attached. Reading labels is essential for people taking insulin to cover what we eat. But when people with diabetes read labels, they often look for sugar content. Checking for sugar on a label is not enough. All carbohydrates (excluding a little fiber) turn into sugar. Sugar is indented under carbs because it is only part of total carbohydrates. The 2019 Nutrition Facts Label I use for teaching shows 12 grams of sugar in one serving, and 37 grams of carbohydrate. If I based my insulin intake on the sugar in that food rather than the carbs I would underestimate and probably end up with high blood sugar. Get good at reading labels on packaged foods, looking online, or using your carb gram counter to find the *total carbohydrates* in the foods you eat.

So-Called Sugar Free Foods!

Most type 1s know that other ingredients in foods designated *sugar free* affect our blood sugar. When I visited my aunt, she offered me sugar-free cookies that she had made especially for her type 1 daughter. They were oatmeal cookies with raisins. Oatmeal, flour and raisins would raise my blood sugar. But my aunt was so pleased that they were sugar free. I didn't explain. It's a balance. They were a better choice with no sugar added. But they were still going to raise my blood sugar.

More upsetting, manufacturers can advertise their products as sugar free, although they include other sweeteners that raise blood sugar, like corn syrup or fructose or molasses or honey. Looking in a pharmacy for gifts for Valentine's Day I saw two candy displays side-by-side. One was labeled sugar free. When I checked labels, the *sugar-free* candies had 25 carb grams in 3 pieces and the ones with sugar had 14 grams in 3 pieces. Damn those manufacturers. Those sugar-free choices would have raised your blood sugar higher than the sugared ones. Unfortunately, people with diabetes assume that sugar-free is a good choice. My dad was thrilled to buy a bag of sugar-free candies, and thought he could eat them all! Just being without sugar isn't enough. Check the carbs.

Sugar Substitutes

Many people with diabetes avoid sugar entirely and instead use sugar substitutes. There are healthy alternatives to sugar. But I do not use or recommend man-made chemical sweeteners. Although the FDA has approved several, and they have been intensively studied, doubts remain about their safety.

If you find the pink, blue or yellow packaged ones helpful and want to continue with them I have been advised not to use too much of any one kind. Alternate them. And be careful not to ingest too much. Clients have told me they stopped drinking sugared sodas but were consuming as much as two six-packs of diet soda in a day! That's way too much sugar substitute and not a healthy habit for other reasons.

Some people who want to avoid sugar think stevia or xylitol are better choices. Stevia is a natural product. When my diabetes educator Paula was a child in South America, stevia grew in neighborhood yards like a weed and was considered poor people's sugar. By itself stevia may be a good choice. However, stevia packets on many grocery store shelves include other ingredients, so check labels.

My cholesterol-lowering non-diabetic friend Helen is committed to avoiding sugar entirely. She employs xylitol and is surprised that I do not. Xylitol is a sugar alcohol, and sugar alcohols send me directly to the toilet. WebMD.com—a trustworthy online source—addresses sugar alcohols and states that, "Xylitol is a naturally occurring alcohol found in most plant material, including many fruits and vegetables." But they warn that xylitol may also be created in a laboratory and can be toxic to dogs! Make sure your xylitol is naturally derived and that your dog doesn't grab one of the sugar-free cookies you just baked! WebMD also reports that sugar alcohols are carbohydrates and can still raise blood sugar, plus they may produce laxative or other digestive symptoms.

Honey and maple syrup are very sweet liquid sugars. Other sweet choices with varying amounts of carbohydrate include monk fruit, coconut sugar, molasses and date sugar. Agave syrup was briefly touted as a good choice for those concerned with blood sugar. But it is a high fructose sweetener said to worsen liver health and reduce insulin sensitivity. That's why agave is no longer considered a good alternative to sugar for people with diabetes.

Medical News Today sums it up:

> People who are following a healthful diet to manage diabetes should reduce their sugar intake rather than switching one type of sugar for another.

That article suggests that we use fruit for extra sweetness. Try using apples or apple sauce as healthy sweeteners for cooking and baking,

How Many Carbs?

One portion of carbohydrates is 15 grams. Now that individualization is so strongly advised, it is hard to find a recommendation for how many carb portions we should consume at one time or in a day. My own diabetes educator says I limit carbohydrates. I didn't realize I was doing that, but it works for me. And it all depends. I have a small frame and don't need much basal insulin. I build more carbs into my meal plan when I'm athletic, or on vacation. I need fewer when I'm sedentary or ill. Find out what works for you!

When I educate women with diabetes, I generally recommend 1-2 carb portions for a snack and 3-4 carb portions for a meal. For a man I recommend 4-5 carb portions for meals and the same 1-2 carb portions for a snack.

The dietitian in my health center's diabetes program offers his clients a broader range of carb portions. (Know too that labels provide information for a serving, which may be different from a carb portion.)

Think of your carb portions as if they were a budget. You have a certain number of carb grams you plan to spend on what you eat and drink at that time. On my plan, you can spend 15-30 grams on a snack and 45-60 grams for women or 60-75 grams for men on a meal. Find out if that's enough for you or too much. Try different amounts and see what works best. Check your blood sugar before you eat to see whether you are in goal range or need to cover a high. Take your insulin, and two hours after your first bite, check your blood sugar again. The recommended 2-hour post-meal blood sugar goal is *lower than 180*.

For building your carb awareness, consider purchasing a carb gram counter. I use the *CalorieKing Calorie, Fat & Carbohydrate Counter*. It is an almost-300-page booklet updated annually that lists foods in alphabetical order and choices at restaurant chains across the United States. (They have a large-print booklet and an app too.)

I gave a copy of the *CalorieKing* counter to a nurse I work with and she went directly to the McDonald's page to find out how many carbs were in her favorite treat. She said a very bad word when she discovered that a 16-ounce McDonald's chocolate shake contains 104 grams of carbohydrate! Divide 104 grams by 15 grams in one portion. The result is 6.93333333 carb portions in that milkshake. She found a different treat.

Using a gram counter or reading labels builds your awareness and helps you make good choices. Counting carbohydrates inevitably reveals that particular foods and drinks we like a lot or consider healthy are also carb rich.

According to *CalorieKing*:

- an average fruit smoothie has 50 grams of carb

- one Starbuck's 8-grain roll has 70 grams of carb

- ¾ cup of Trader Joe's low fat granola has 44 grams of carb (and that doesn't include the milk you put on it)

Making good choices is tricky. At Starbuck's I can drink a cup of coffee with half-and-half that has 0 carbs. But a small Mocha adds up to 48 grams—3+ portions.

Having an idea how many carbs my favorite foods contain is very satisfying. My workplace carb portion handout tells me that 12 fresh cherries—which I love—are one serving of carbohydrate. When I toured the Flathead Lake orchards in Montana during cherry season, fruit was on sale everywhere. I could buy a bag of cherries, sit on a stone fence and confidently count 12-24 cherries into my mouth for a snack, take my insulin and know that my blood sugar would respond well.

On that trip I also encountered huckleberries in pie and syrup in restaurants. I know that generally a cup of berries is a portion, but I wasn't sure how much sugar had been added to huckleberry pie or syrup, so I left those alone. I was on a pleasure trip and didn't want to trouble my journey with high or low blood sugar after trying to cover those unknowns. I stuck to what I knew. When I got home, I looked in my gram counter and found that a small piece of berry pie has 49 carb grams, and ¼ cup of fruit syrup has 52 carb grams. Glad I skipped them.

Tips for Handling Carbs

- Learn how many carbs are in your favorite or everyday foods.

- Fill your kitchen with low-carb foods that are satisfying and provide balance.

- Switch to open-face sandwiches. Pile your one piece of bread with meat or cheese and top with lettuce or spinach or kale or basil.

- When you buy a sandwich or burger toss away half the bun or ask your waiter to wrap your burger in lettuce.

- Measure out snacks instead of eating straight from the bag or box.

- Limit seconds unless it's more vegetables or protein.

- Partner your carbohydrates with protein or fat to help keep blood sugar from spiking and to make meals more satisfying.

- Call yourself a picky eater. Pick the foods that serve you best and are delicious.

- Travelers, do your prep work. Before hitting Europe or Asia or the state next door, find out what people eat, what you might want to try, and be prepared. Even in our own country there are major differences. Are you ready to encounter Montana huckleberry pie, Chicago deep dish pizza, New Mexico sopaipillas with honey, or South Carolina sweet tea?

Diabetes has helped me find a way of eating that nurtures me and is enjoyable. I choose high quality delicious food, often made by me at home. Both my taste buds and my belly are happy.

What if you don't cook?

- Play with frozen or canned foods.

- Open a can of tomatoes and a can of beans. Pour them into a saucepan with water or stock. Add onion powder, garlic powder and dried oregano. You have soup!

- Fill your freezer with frozen vegetables when they are on sale. Shake a serving of veggies into your scrambled eggs.

- Buy fresh already-washed spinach and drop a handful on a hot plate of enchiladas or a bowl of stew. The spinach will be steamed on the way to your table. (I discovered this at *El Sombrero* café in Socorro, New Mexico.)

- Turn a pre-mixed salad into a feast with chickpeas, olives, good cheese, avocado, and a hard-boiled egg or tuna.

Can't resist cookies, pretzels, chips? Stock your cupboards with lower-carb treats. Or go ahead with your cravings every now and then, cover them with insulin and see what happens! When I was diagnosed with celiac disease I went through a must-have-pretzels stage. I ate boxes and bags of gluten-free pretzels made primarily with corn meal, taking plenty of insulin so my blood sugar didn't go crazy. Finally, I had enough. They tasted like dust in my mouth and I moved on.

Experts consider a few foods addictive, or think because we crave them we are addicted. I've been told that various companies do include ingredients that may cause addiction. And sugar has that reputation. I don't like the label *addiction* because it appears to leave out choice. Most of us can choose what we eat and drink and how much. And my own experience is that denying myself something makes me want it more. I carefully allow a version of my cravings until they are satisfied. I have friends who say they cannot have cookies in the house because they will eat them all. One type 1 I know could not keep hard candies at home for hypo times because she would devour even those. Nurture yourself in other ways so food rewards are less important.

Novel Approaches

As I explained with pretzels, one of my discoveries is that when I give myself what I want, after a while I no longer crave it. At a certain point, probably around Halloween, I desperately craved Snickers bars. I bought an original 1.9 ounce Snickers bar, 33 grams of carb. I took my insulin, cut the Snickers bar lengthwise and then into bite-size pieces. I placed the pieces on a lovely gilded plate, ate it with a fork and savored every bite. I repeated that ritual once more and haven't wanted to eat Snickers since. Reminds me that a doc told me, "No one should eat dessert every day and neither should you." No one should eat Snickers every day and neither should I. But saying, "Never!" makes me want it more.

My overall method, which I teach my clients, is to eat the carbs you like the best and let the others wait for another time. Selecting my favorite carbs on Thanksgiving Day I want mashed potatoes with gravy, a bite of sweet potatoes, and peas. I skip sweet drinks, fruit salad, rolls or bread, and stuffing. With plenty of turkey and a green salad or broccoli, I am set. After dinner I take a walk, and a couple of hours later enjoy pumpkin pie. Whipped cream is great without added sugar, and it serves me better than ice cream with my pie. I can eat both carefully and sumptuously on holidays.

Start by savoring whatever you are eating. Slow down and thank your body for using your food in a heathy way. Another wise step is to bring to a gathering what you like and know you can handle. I often prepare dessert for a potluck because I can identify exactly what's in it and how much is good for me.

Another of my tips is to stock your kitchen with appealing low-carb snacks. Some of my favorites are:

- Roasted pumpkin seeds, plain or spicy

- Cottage cheese or plain yogurt topped with salsa and chopped nuts

- Marinated mushrooms or artichoke hearts in half a bell pepper or scooped-out cucumber

- Salami and cheese wrapped in lettuce leaves

- Half an avocado with salsa in the middle

- Cucumber or zucchini sliced in rounds to replace chips (You up your vegetable intake and can scoop guacamole or hummus or salsa.)

Alcohol

Alcoholic beverages may be controversial for people with diabetes. For those who feel comfortable drinking alcohol, the American Diabetes Association holds the same alcohol standard for people with diabetes as for any others: No more than one drink per day for women and no more than two for men.

Alcohol in combination with type 1 diabetes is complicated because your liver is affected. Also difficult is that different types of alcoholic beverages have varied carb counts. Many people mistakenly believe that alcohol is sweet. It is not particularly sweet because sugar is consumed in the process of creating alcohol.

Remember that 15 grams of carbohydrate equals one portion. A 6-ounce glass of wine, either red or white, averages 5 grams of carb. Hard liquor has zero carbs. The carbs are in the mix. For example, a shot of tequila has no carbs. But a margarita has 29 grams. Beer carb counts vary from light beer at 4 carb grams per 7-ounce glass, to 30 grams or more in a craft beer, so it's best to look up your favorite.

Essential for those with diabetes is to eat when you drink alcohol. Otherwise you may get hypoglycemic. Ordinarily your liver sends out sugar to cover lows. But when you drink alcoholic beverages your liver is occupied with clearing alcohol from your body. Hypoglycemia may sneak up on you, symptoms hidden by the effects of alcohol.

For parties and other outings where you will consume alcohol, consider bringing along a companion who can help if your blood sugar goes dangerously low. Also know that the effects of alcohol on your blood sugar may continue into the next day. Keep track.

Remember

- Carbohydrates raise blood sugar.

- Know what you are eating.

- Find the right kind of advice.

- Learn more.

- Eat to create satisfaction and overall glowing health.

- Your taste buds will become more sensitive and you will become more discerning.

- Check blood sugar before and after questionable meals so you know what works and doesn't. Dietitians recommend keeping a food journal for a few days and comparing what you eat and drink with your blood sugar results.

- Discover what eating plan works for your blood sugar, lifestyle and happiness and stick to it!

Food is our survival and also a source of comfort and contentment. Most of us most of the time are fortunate to have enough food and many choices. Find your own way to eat what keeps your blood sugar steady and feeds you on all levels—body, mind, heart and soul. That's probably a lifetime quest.

All you need is love. But a little chocolate now and then doesn't hurt.

Charles M. Schulz
Cartoonist and Creator of the Comic Strip *Peanuts*

CHAPTER 13

Keep Moving

One of the most important ways we can and must take care of ourselves is to keep moving. Staying physically active is essential for every human and absolutely vital for type 1s. Besides contributing to our overall bodily health, exercise helps us manage our blood sugar and prevent the long-term complications we want to avoid. The American Psychological Association states that exercise of any type is beneficial for mental health as well as physical health. Physical activity supports our bodies, our minds and our emotions, making it easier to do all we need to do to handle our conditions.

What are we supposed to do?

Based on the results of the Diabetes Prevention Program (1996-2001), adults with diabetes are encouraged to spend *at least* 150 minutes a week being active. That equates to 30 minutes of exercise five days a week. It may be helpful to know that 30 minutes a day can be broken down into smaller segments, for example, 10 minutes of physical activity three times a day.

Whatever you're doing you can find a way to be more active. You know a few tricks: park your car on the far side of the lot, take the stairs, rise from your desk and walk around. For my clients working at home making jewelry, I recommend unfolding from their curled-over positions hammering silver or setting stones, and taking 10-minute breaks to stretch and move.

If glued to a computer, you are advised to rest your eyes by looking out a window and taking the long view. Walk and stretch while you adjust your eyesight.

Set a timer for breaks. Notice how your body feels when you tune in. When I quit reading or writing and stand up, I am always surprised to find myself stiff and awkward at first. Maybe my body was made to move, but I do not always listen to that wisdom. A quick exercise break loosens my muscles and sends me back to my work refreshed.

When building in regular exercise, walking and stretching are obvious choices for most of us because they can be done anywhere, anytime and cost nothing. One of the MDs I work with gardens till dark, then cooks dinner and watches television. She stands up and marches during commercials when she watches TV. I could do that. Or I could finish dinner, join friends or family members and take a walk.

The benefits of exercise cannot be argued. Being active lifts your spirits, clarifies your thinking and tones your body—no matter how you do it. And it can be experienced for free! How come it's so hard? Why are so many of us avoiding regular exercise, especially when we know how important it is for preventing complications of diabetes and ageing?

Numerous studies and surveys reveal that about half of Americans don't meet recommended activity guidelines. Half of us! Researchers suggest that our commitment to being active or not is influenced by family and cultural attitudes, and even the neighborhoods we grew up in.

Take a moment to look back at what has affected your attitudes about physical activity.

- Were you encouraged to be active as a child?

- Were your parents or siblings or friends energetic?

- How fun was it to run or bike or skateboard or swim?

- Were you on a school team?

- Did you set physical goals for yourself?

- Were the children of your religion or culture physically active?

- Was your neighborhood safe?

When I was 12, I lived in a suburb of Charleston, South Carolina. After school my mother ordered me and my sisters to change clothes and "Go outside and play!" My best friends Tina and Paula and I hula hooped for hours, talking nonstop while we circled our safe neighborhood. Together we entered a local contest and all three of us won bicycles for continuing to spin those hoops for 12 hours! I could not and would not have done that alone. I was just fortunate to have a mother who pushed me out the door and two determined friends who stuck with me to reach a monumental goal. Now I have to create exercise goals for myself.

Inspirational encounters help. Recently I worked with a client with type 2 diabetes who had already walked 9,500 steps before we met at 10 a.m. Evelyn revealed that she loved walking. But over several weeks she had only lost two pounds, and losing weight was a primary goal for her activity. Briefly devastated by that *failure* she stopped walking. In conversation with her medical provider she realized that her clothes were fitting more loosely and she was building muscle. Although she was not losing weight, walking was reshaping her body. With that awareness, Evelyn returned to walking with even greater intensity. She showed me her Fitbit reports on steps completed that week by herself, her walking partner, and friends and family members. Those Fitbit reports encouraged her and her cadre to take on new goals. And her enthusiasm inspired me to extend my daily walks.

- Are you active every single day?

- Are you pleased with what you've chosen to do?

- Does your physical activity leave you feeling better when finished than you did when you started?

- What gets you going and keeps you moving?

Let your thoughts aid you in building or enhancing an exercise plan that perfectly fits you. If you don't know what your exercise priority is yet, be curious. Try new things. A woman I work with turned 50 and was invited to meet friends at a lake and try paddle boarding. Even when dumped into cold water again and again, she enjoyed herself so much that she bought a board. Now she puts everything else aside to get back to the lake and onto her paddle board.

Type 1 doesn't stop you!

Having type 1 diabetes does not keep us from any physical activity. Type 1s are marathon runners and professional football, hockey and baseball players. We are Olympic medalists and ordinary people playing golf or tennis or catch with our kids in the back yard. Type 1 is no reason to stop intense activity that you love. Nor is it a reason to avoid taking on a physical challenge that interests you.

Some of us have to move. It's part of us, part of how we express ourselves or nurture ourselves or stay sane. As a young woman I took an Outward Bound wilderness course and then spent a decade hiking and climbing and leading others through jubilant and terrifying mountain experiences. Looking back now I am sure that those wilderness adventures kept my blood sugar in control and protected me in the time before rapid-acting insulin and glucose meters. Vibrantly healthy in body and mind, I adored being able to hike for miles through wild places carrying everything I needed on my back. Unfortunately, I have grown more sedentary with time.

With luck, being active is an expression of your true self. You may already be a runner, a skier, a hang glider, a swimmer, a mountain climber, a speed walker, or a dancer. You have found what works for you and moved into it.

But some of us do *not* love to exercise. Nor do we have a life goal that demands physical strength and stamina. We may even hate to exercise. Is that you? Do you want to skip this chapter because it makes you feel like a failure from the start? Even if this topic is dreadful, give it careful thought. You do not have to be anyone else's idea of an athlete. Finding the right exercise is satisfyingly individual. With investigation you will find there are ways that your body would like to move.

My friend Ava has discovered Qi Gong. She tried many movement specialties and nothing else made it easy for her to continue. She loves doing Qi Gong and says that's because one movement is slowly repeated many times so she can settle in without memorizing or thinking about her routine. She is able to flow.

How might you build in greater physical activity, reap the benefits, and be encouraged rather than discouraged? What physical activity is compelling and practical enough for you to turn into a habit? Like everything else about type 1 diabetes, it depends.

Exercise might bring out the best or the worst in you, probably both at one time or another. When the switchbacks to that mountain pass are cramping my calves and blistering my heels, why do I keep going? I want to have lunch where I can see the other side! So I curse and stomp and walk a little farther.

When it's a blizzardy zero degrees and time to take a walk, what gets me out the door? I am stiff and knotted up from hunching over my laptop. I have a cat on my lap. My mind is locked on repetitive thoughts. I need to get outside and appreciate my surroundings. I remind myself that I want to stay strong. I know my mind will clear and I will feel more creative. I let myself complain while I put on warm clothes and supportive shoes. But I get ready and go! I start walking, congratulate myself and laugh at my stubbornness. Appreciation and a sense of humor motivate me.

You and I who are not natural athletes have to create exercise plans we can do, we want to do, and we can stick with. We proceed through trial and error to find the right activity at the right time. Here are examples of what has and hasn't worked for me.

Years ago I decided to adopt a dog who would force me to get out and walk. My friend Dawna walks everywhere, squired by her two dogs, and I wanted that for myself. But a pregnant cat showed up at my door, so I stayed home and raised kittens. Not a good exercise plan.

For several years I met weekly for a private Pilates lesson with a wonderful instructor. I started each class feeling grumpy. After an hour guided firmly but laughingly through Pilates movements I was smiling and moving more comfortably. I liked my instructor. I felt better after our sessions. I made a financial investment in my health and didn't want to waste my money, so I never missed a class! All that worked for me.

Pushing me to stay active between classes, my Pilates instructor gave me stretch moves to do on a large fitness ball. I bought a ball, brought it home and inflated it. But I didn't do those stretches. After months kicking the ball out of the way in my small house, I admitted that I would never use it. I deflated the ball and stashed it in my junk room. That plan never worked.

When my Pilates teacher moved away, I signed up with another instructor who came highly recommended, and took classes with her for several months. Finally I gave myself permission to quit. Although she was a kind and knowledgeable instructor, she was an academic and wanted me to understand the movements and their results. I just wanted to move. The sessions she led me through didn't satisfy my body or my emotions. I left each class disgruntled and unsatisfied. That was not a good plan for me.

During the Covid-19 crisis I was invited to free online yoga classes several times a week. When I attended, I hated the classes and quit before the end. I could not manage most of the poses and was told that I would improve and must just start. I have *just started* yoga many times over the years and still hate it. I once pulled off the road to cry on the way to a yoga class, knowing I could never do a creditable forward bend. Not a good exercise plan for me.

Fortunately, I can participate fully in Classical Stretch classes with Miranda Esmonde-White, who leads sessions on my Public Broadcasting Service TV station. Esmonde-White is in her 70s and wrote the book *Aging Backwards*. She models poses I can copy at my level of fitness, and I can discern improvement as I continue. Hurray! This works.

As you find the right form of exercise and advance, be aware that both your willingness and your physical abilities may change over time. MD Andrew Weil wrote *Healthy Aging: A Lifelong Guide to Your Physical and Spiritual Well-Being*, and rebuilt his practice around healthy aging.

It helped me to hear Weil describe the emotions he went through when his body demanded that he stop running. Now he swims laps.

Although I was once a mountaineer and walked many miles a day for weeks at a time, today I struggle to stay active. When I get out the door in my small city, I love to walk, which is great exercise and works for my body. But getting out that door is often difficult. I am seduced by the comfort of another cup of coffee or an Internet search or a good book or my next writing project, so walking is postponed.

Set a life goal.

My recommendation for establishing and maintaining an enjoyable and effective physical routine is to base it on a personal goal. Consider what you like to do that would benefit from building strength or endurance.

Some type 1s start walking with a plan to take part in the annual *Walk for Diabetes*. Others get excited about completing a 5k or 10k race or even a marathon, and work with a coach or a circle of friends to train for that goal. Maybe you plan a tour of famous European sites and want to be able to walk all day. Or you want to trek to Machu Picchu, or take your grandchildren to a beach to snorkel and surf. Your goal may even be simpler: you want to carry your groceries up the stairs to your third-floor apartment without gasping for breath.

Whatever your life goal, being strong and agile will help you. What adventure do you have in mind that calls for greater muscle and stamina?

With a compelling goal, make an exercise plan. You may be able to bike to work or to the grocery store. You may join an online class where you have music and companions from around the world exercising alongside you. You and your partner may dance together and feel better and happier as you express yourselves.

Sometimes knowing whether you are introverted or extroverted helps. I hated going to a gym when I tried it, and don't even want to join friends exercising on Zoom. I would rather walk or take a recorded class in my home alone. My walking client Evelyn is more extroverted. She depends on her walking partner—who texts to wake her up on the mornings they go walking. Both introverted and extroverted friends of mine have turned their garages into workout rooms or their backyards into physical challenge courses. Embrace your possibilities. Create a plan that's both achievable and satisfying.

And anytime you resist completing your daily exercise commitment, remind yourself that you want to be healthy and able to easily make your goals come true. When I am postponing or lagging on my walks I tell myself that walking keeps me strong. It does. I want to stay strong, so I keep going. My current goal is a trek in the Colorado Rockies, and I don't want to drag along huffing and puffing behind my companions. I need to establish a routine and discover how to stabilize my blood sugar. I most certainly do not want to bring on either hypo- or hyperglycemic episodes. Therefore I keep walking.

Blood sugar changes with exercise.

Diabetes educators have demonstrated the benefits of exercise for type 2s by feeding them a high carb breakfast and then putting them on treadmills. Blood sugar is checked before and after exercise and clearly comes down. Exercise parameters for type 1s are more complicated.

The British medical journal *Lancet* published a 2017 consensus statement on exercise management for T1Ds.

> Regular physical activity should be a routine objective for patients with type 1 diabetes, for various health and fitness reasons…. In general, aerobic exercise is associated with reductions in glycaemia, whereas anaerobic exercise might be associated with a transient increase in glucose concentrations. Both forms of exercise can cause delayed-onset hypoglycaemia in recovery….

Aerobic exercise is known as *cardio* and includes activities like brisk walking, swimming, running, or cycling. During aerobic exercise you breathe harder, your heart rate increases and you build endurance. Overall, it's aerobic exercise that burns glucose and sends your blood sugar low.

Anaerobic exercise, such as weightlifting, jumping rope or sprinting, involves bursts of energy for a short time to promote bone and muscle strength. Anaerobic exercise might temporarily raise your blood sugar. It uses sugar stored in the muscles as glycogen and may produce adrenaline. As a reaction to those hormones your liver might try to compensate by adding more sugar to your blood.

Be aware that hypoglycemia from either form of exercise can occur during or long after an exercise session. Blood sugar lowered by exercise may remain low over a surprising length of time—for hours or even into the next day.

Knowing how to adjust your carb intake and insulin rate for particular physical activities is essential. For aerobic exercise you may need to stave off hypoglycemia by lowering your insulin dose or increasing carb intake before, during and after your exercise session. Anaerobic activities may not require any insulin adjustment or greater carb intake. But after anaerobic exercise, monitor your blood sugar carefully to address highs or lows. And be aware that often the two types of exercise are intertwined. Stay in touch with your beautifully active body.

Reviewing your exercise plans with your health team may be helpful. And remember that no matter what guidelines are recommended, you have to find your own way. You will never know where an exercise plan will take you until you try it, so venture into new activities carefully. Once you experience how your body reacts to certain exercises, you can experiment more confidently.

Goals again...

If you are not naturally athletic, you may not yet have a goal or a passion that encourages you to be active. And you may not know what walking or running or weightlifting or getting on a paddle board will do to your blood sugar. African American television show writer, producer and director Shonda Rhimes offers advice about life that applies to your exercise goals and workout experiments.

> Maybe you know exactly what it is you dream of being, or maybe you're paralyzed because you have no idea what your passion is. The truth is that it doesn't matter. You don't have to know. You just have to keep moving forward. You just have to keep doing something, seizing the next opportunity, staying open to trying something new.

You don't have to know what you are exercising for. Just keep moving forward. Try something new. Be prepared. Track the blood sugar lowering effects of aerobic exercise, or increasing effects of anaerobic exercise. Make adjustments for potential hypo, immediately and/or many hours after you work out. A walk, even a brisk walk, may or may not bring on hypoglycemia. An hour-long yoga class may cause high or low blood sugar. There are numerous possibilities. You are an individual. You need to discover how your body responds and establish appropriate methods for addressing your needs. The extra effort is worth it. You will be liberated. As Nike encourages, "Just do it!"

Keep reading for ideas on how to start.

CHAPTER 14

Starting Your Exercise Program

Engaging in the recommended 150 minutes or more of moderate-to-vigorous aerobic activity per week, and including strength-building anaerobic exercise—is a fulfilling but challenging commitment. You are also urged to decrease the amount of time you are sedentary.

In an April 2020 Public Broadcasting Service episode entitled "Blood Sugar Rising," the narrator declared that we live in a world that is made for type 2 diabetes. With the awareness that only about half of Americans meet recommended activity guidelines, and one night's evaluation of food commercials on TV, it is easy to see how that conclusion was reached.

Onset of type 2 is related to lifestyle. And although type 1 diabetes is not brought on by poor lifestyle, our habits after diagnosis clearly matter. When we are sedentary and eat badly our health declines.

- What might lift you out of the inactive pool of Americans into an active lifestyle?

- How do you make yourself engage in exercise you aren't quite sure you want to do?

Although you desire the positive effects that exercise offers, finding the right form of activity and discovering how to keep your blood sugar steady in response to exercise isn't easy. It might take any number of personal attributes considered positive or negative, to get started and keep going. You might employ willpower, self-discipline, self-mastery, compromise, bargaining, or even coercion, resistance, denial, etc. Counter-reaction has been helpful to me. Tell me I can't and I'll prove you wrong by doing it!

I was diagnosed with type 1 at age 14 and from time to time I still have to negotiate with that balky teen within me. I tell my clients, and I tell you, do what you can to comfort and nurture your child within. If staying active seems too hard, find a way to be an encouraging parent for your inner child. Apply all your skills to inspire a resistant part of yourself to include regular exercise. And remember that making physical activity fun helps. I didn't hula hoop for 12 hours because I knew it was good for me.

It takes self-awareness and commitment to come up with a plan and get yourself ready to start. It takes further commitment to continue exercising each day once you have begun. Find your motivation. Put exercise on your *Top 10 Life List*. Make it satisfying. Results will show up quickly in your mood and energy levels as well as your blood sugar. Keep yourself safe and step into it.

The key is to select an activity you like to do and build it into your daily routine. Find ways to increase both strength and flexibility. Maybe you will take steps on your own. Or, since exercise benefits all, maybe you will involve your family or friends. Christine loves music and dances around her home with her grandchildren. Alan walks with his spouse. They wear pedometers and challenge each other to go farther, laughing and talking as they end their day with movement. Trish adores spinning with her Zoom adversaries. She is on her own but can apply her competitive nature. And Mark is a firefighter who runs with his teammates between shifts.

You are advised to start any exercise plan with a comprehensive health screening. Then begin slowly and intensify as you progress. Call on the member of your health care team most likely to have expertise with physical activity. Or ask for referrals. If you have a specific and challenging plan ahead, like going from not running at all to participating in a 5k run, you might add a physical fitness expert to your team.

Neither my endocrinologist nor my primary doc would be helpful with specifics about my physical activity. But my diabetes educator would remind me how to set a temporary basal rate on my insulin pump and when to add extra carbs. And a fitness instructor would have specific ideas on building my strength for a trek.

Finding *Your* Way

Be wise about your own needs and abilities. Although type 1 diabetes doesn't stop you, it has to be carefully managed. Fear of blood sugar consequences may rightfully hold you back. Passing out due to hypo, or rising dangerously high, are extreme examples of where your blood sugar might take you in response to exercise. No need to go there. Be a detective and discover your body's response to your exercise plan.

To fortify your plan, you might enlist team members and gather information from books or articles or blogs written by type 1 athletes. Being active is a high priority for your health. You can be both creative and sensible about your abilities, and get support if you need it.

Once you have an idea what you'd like to do, determine how to start from where you are. Perhaps you want to hike the 26-mile Inca Trail at high altitude to Machu Picchu in six months. But you cannot currently walk a mile in your sea-level neighborhood. You need to start slowly and carefully and stick with your strength- and stamina-building commitment. You probably need expert advice and support. And you will build experience as you put your plan into action.

The American Diabetes Association urges type 1s to plan ahead for exercise, and to check blood sugar before, during and after exercise to see how it's affecting you, especially when doing something new.

Start exercising with your blood sugar in goal range and pay attention to what it does as you continue. Keep track. Apply your results to customize your insulin dose and food choices for future activity. Your diabetes goal is to avoid highs or lows and keep your blood sugar steady. (Remember that most types of insulin take a while to act. Adjusting insulin before you begin to exercise may help.)

As your body changes in response to regular exercise, your insulin and carb needs may change again and again. With experience you will become your own expert advisor. Part of the gift of diabetes is to be in touch with your body and build your ability to recognize its signals. Tune in to what your body is telling you. Don't rush past physical sensations. Notice them and reassure your body. I have a right ankle that periodically pains me. Halfway through my daily walk it may speak up. I walk more slowly, breathe through the pain, and thank that ankle for all it does for me. Sometimes the pain dissipates and sometimes it doesn't. Depending on my ankle's response I may continue on my intended route. Or I may slow my pace and shorten my walk.

Professional athletes have different ways of addressing such challenges, but are generally solidly in touch with their bodies. The internet has a number of reputable blog sites by and for people with type 1 diabetes. And three magazines I receive, *Diabetes Forecast*, *Diabetes Self-Management* and *Diabetic Living* all introduce heroes, heroines and ordinary people who speak about their lives with T1D. Enjoy finding an athlete whose story inspires your diabetes exercise world. Find out how they became athletic and how they stay in shape.

Remember to breathe! Athletes and their coaches pay attention to breathing and so do meditation teachers! Breathing feeds our bodies as they activate and it also soothes us when we slow and become aware of our breath. I teach my clients with diabetes the simplest stress-reducing technique—three deep breaths slowly in and out.

Besides determining your physical capacity as a person with type 1 diabetes, you are honing your ability to tune in, think clearly, make plans and respond accurately. You are inviting your diabetes to educate and support you.

Fine Tuning

Experts warn that there are times type 1s should not exercise. If your blood sugar is 270 mg/dL or higher when you are preparing for an exercise class or session, check for ketones. Exercising when ketones are present could send your blood sugar dangerously high, so you are urged to postpone activity and take steps to bring your blood sugar back to normal.

Consider what time of day works best for you to exercise and create a regular workout schedule. I do best at walking or taking my stretch class first thing in the morning. Before walking I check my CGM for blood sugar level, make sure my carb fix is in my pocket and walk at a steady pace for an hour. Walking is aerobic, so I watch out for low blood sugar during and after.

My stretching/strengthening class is anaerobic and sends my blood sugar up. But it is only 30 minutes long so I do not make special adjustments. I start at about 120 mg/dL without eating, and am usually in the 180s when finished. I program an insulin correction and have a cup of coffee, giving my body time to return to my goal blood sugar before eating. Since I exercise early, I can keep track of my blood sugar all day, and am less likely to go too low while asleep.

Every person is unique. You won't know how your body responds to exercise until you try new routines yourself. You may apply aspects of what I have suggested or follow expert advice and still need to adjust. And you will change. Life circumstances, age, recovering from surgery or injury, life stresses, even your mood, all affect your body's responses to your exercise plan.

First and foremost, find out what inspires you. Try new movements that you have wondered about. Once begun stay curious. Continue adjusting your exercise program to keep you happy and growing. You are moving for a handful of good reasons and are building a deeper relationship with your diabetes.

Some keep a journal that illustrates their progress. Others use a pedometer or a Fitbit or an app that helps them track their development and blood sugar results. Create and alter your plans as needed. Be prepared for high or low blood sugar and ready to treat it. When you have established a routine, celebrate your results and rejoice in your willingness to incorporate movement into your busy and fulfilling life. Keep exploring to find your way.

When it comes to health and well-being, regular exercise is about as close to a magic potion as you can get.

Tich Nhat Hanh, age 94
Buddhist Monk and Peace Activist

CHAPTER 15

Wake Up! Sleep Matters

When I began writing this chapter I was astonished at where it took me. I had not realized that both individuals and providers usually slide right past the topic of sleep. Although vital to your health, sleep is not always considered in the medical world. Prepare to be enlightened.

My friend Sue falls into bed at night with a smile. "Bed," she croons, "sleep." She has found the perfect time to go to sleep, knows how many hours of sleep support her, and has made a commitment to her good sleep habits.

Knowing that I am not so good about sleeping well, I envy her. I have no sleep routine. I stay up too long. I watch the late night show while playing word games on my computer, not wearing the recommended glasses that filter blue screen light. Although I stop caffeine at noon, I eat or drink anything else till bedtime.

Once I set my alarm—often indicating too few hours to sleep—I fall into bed exhausted. My two cats are clamped to either side of me, purring. I am wrapped like a burrito and dare not roll over. They will wake me at 6 a.m. to feed them. On a workday I stay up and get underway. On off days I feed the cats and stumble back to bed.

Although my bedroom is dark, I bring in screen light—checking my CGM results on my phone, which, with my insulin pump, will send blood sugar alerts during the night. I prop my iPad against my pillow and direct it to read to me. ALL WRONG!

My sleep habits are worst on the nights before I go to work. I suspect my teenaged inner self takes charge and pushes me to resist what I *ought* to do. Next morning I struggle to rise, curse my schedule, and discover that my blood sugar sat steadily high at 170 all night. Looking in the bathroom mirror I hope my glasses will hide the circles under my eyes. Throughout the day I take deep breaths to oxygenate my failing brain, and vow to do better. I comfort myself that I will *catch up* on sleep over the weekend. But experts don't think we can catch up.

You may be doing everything right and sleeping like an angel. If so, I salute you and invite you to congratulate yourself. You may not even want to read this! But I have added this consequential chapter because sleep is an essential nurturing asset to our lives as humans and as humans with type 1 diabetes. If you aren't sleeping well, perhaps this information will inspire you to enrich your sleep life.

Shouldn't sleeping well be automatic? Unfortunately, like everything else about our health with type 1 diabetes, getting proper sleep takes a number of possibly difficult steps. And we need good sleep even more than most people.

Poor quality sleep affects your glycemic control and increases your risk of complications. Some think sleep affects everything: metabolism, appetite, cravings, and hormones including insulin. And sleep disturbance is a circle. Your blood sugar, blood pressure and diabetes affect your sleep and your sleep affects your blood sugar, blood pressure and diabetes.

Camille Peri quoted sleep specialists and studies for her article, "10 Things to Hate About Sleep Loss" for WebMD. Peri wrote:

1. Sleepiness causes accidents.

2. Sleep loss dumbs you down.

3. Sleep deprivation can lead to serious health problems.

4. Lack of sleep kills sex drive.

5. Sleepiness is depressing.

6. Lack of sleep ages your skin.

7. Sleepiness makes you forgetful.

8. Losing sleep can make you gain weight.

9. Lack of sleep may increase risk of death.

10. Sleep loss impairs judgment, especially about sleep.

On the other hand, in "Surprising Reasons to Get More Sleep" reviewed in 2019, WebMD listed what *good* sleep does for us:

1. Sharper brain

2. Mood boost

3. Healthier heart

4. Athletic achievement

5. Steadier blood sugar

6. Germ fighting

7. Weight control

That article also warns not to sleep too much, which further limits the value of my weekend catch-ups. How can *you* improve your sleep?

—

Barriers to Sleep

Even without medical emphasis, I know that whether we are type 1s or not, better sleep is a tremendous asset. What stops us from insisting on better sleep?

The Sleep Health Foundation lists barriers to good sleep:

- Taking sleep for granted

- Too much caffeine, alcohol and sleeping tablets

- Shift work

- Jet lag

- Eating and drinking late

- Failing to wind down before bed

- Stress

- Sleep disorders

- Other medical conditions and pregnancy

- Drug side effects (over-the-counter or prescription)

I add further barriers:

- Beliefs, for example, "I might miss something," or "I have a late night personality."

- Sharing your household with another adult who stays up late.

- Or—like my mom when her children were small— rising early to have time for yourself.

Realize that humans do not make changes just for health! We need to get personal. If poor sleep worsens my complexion and affects my looks, I might change. If poor sleep means I snap at my spouse or children, I might change. If poor sleep puts me at risk of losing the job I love, I might change, etc.

—

How does this matter to me as a type 1?

One doctor's review of 60 sleep studies showed a consistent rate of 15% or higher sleep problems in type 1s. Some researchers set that number even higher. A 2011 study found that 35% of people with type 1 diabetes sleep poorly.

In February 2016, *Diabetes Spectrum* journal published "Type 1 Diabetes and Sleep." The article concluded that more research is needed to determine why type 1s have higher rates of sleep disturbance and what that means to our overall health.

Experts also believe that people who have had type 1 the longest are at greatest risk. But remember! Diabetes alone is not a risk factor and neither is length of diabetes. Poorly controlled diabetes causes trouble. Bad sleep may be an aspect of poor control. One more hiccup in your diabetes tango! How can *you* improve your sleep?

The article "Type 1 Diabetes and Sleep" provided a surprise for me. It concluded that "lack of the normal decline in blood pressure during sleep may be linked to short sleep duration in people with type 1 diabetes, and this may accelerate the development of cardiovascular and microvascular disease." No medical advisor has ever raised poor sleep as a possible contributor to my high blood pressure or to complications—including threats to my eyesight.

Starting in 2017, the American Diabetes Association recommended including sleep assessment as part of medical evaluations for people with diabetes. Specialists agree that sleep habits should be considered essential topics any MD or CDCES addresses.

Of course doctors and diabetes educators should ask us about our sleep and make recommendations for better sleep. But we mostly don't. Besides the complexity of improving sleep habits, time is an issue for providers and overwhelm is an issue for patients. Fifteen minutes with a doctor may be too little time, and 30-60 minutes with a diabetes educator may be too much! Usually the two appointments are linked, and as a patient I have been known to stagger out of a clinic after two appointments, unable to incorporate all the information put before me.

What can providers and educators do?

First and foremost, many of us in the medical world don't realize that sleep is so important, and don't know what to do about it except to refer patients to a sleep study. And our patients don't realize that their sleep habits affect their diabetes and their overall health and happiness. All of us need a *heads up* on sleep.

Occasionally I ask patients how they are sleeping, but I have never gone deeply into that issue. One of the MDs I work with is very aware and outspoken about sleep. In her work with obese type 2s in particular, Dr. Sullivan regularly diagnoses sleep apnea and helps patients make changes to manage it.

Although I stride into exam rooms with a rolling case of informational files, I had never even looked for a sleep handout until writing this chapter! Thankfully I discovered that my favorite resource, learningaboutdiabetes.org, has a handout titled Diabetes and Sleep. That page offers tips as well as confirming that getting good sleep is important and may be difficult. (Learningaboutdiabetes.org provides colorful low-literacy visual pages on many topics in many languages. Their handouts are free to individuals and can be used by professionals for a small fee.)

There is so much to cover in a traditional medical appointment. Providers need to determine whether patients are taking their medications and whether those medications are doing their jobs. They need to look at A1cs or CGM reports and discuss patients' blood sugar levels. And they must address patients' concerns and fears. When a patient then gets to me, they usually only want to talk about food!

Certainly good eating is important but it's only one aspect of blood sugar control. The Association of Diabetes Care and Education Specialists offers diabetes educators its system of seven self-care behaviors to cover with patients.

They are:

1. Healthy Coping

2. Healthy Eating

3. Being Active

4. Monitoring

5. Taking Medication

6. Problem Solving

7. Reducing Risks

Healthy coping has recently been moved to the top. And sleep would probably come under Reducing Risks—but only if I have time to get past other risks raised by the patient.

Clearly all of the *essential seven* cannot be addressed in one visit. I encourage clients to come back in a month. But follow-up appointments depend on whether the patient considers further diabetes education important, whether their schedule permits, whether their health care insurance will cover visits, and more. Telephone calls or official telemedicine visits are certainly valuable. And they too depend on a patient's interest, availability and technology.

As a diabetes coach I have clients who know that our meetings are of value. We set up a series of talks to address their concerns and track their growth. As a diabetes educator for T2Ds at a health center I am not so fortunate. Wretchedly, I compare my record of returning patients to Lucy at her *psychiatric help 5¢* booth in the *Peanuts* comic strip. Lucy didn't have many takers.

Although I want every client I meet with to sleep better, your health is in your own hands. When you meet with your doctor or your diabetes educator they may not bring up sleep. But you can. As a patient you might get help and also educate the medical world!

Improving Your Sleep

Yes, there are ways you can improve your sleep. Suggestions for a better night's sleep include:

- Establish a regular routine and stick to it.

- Exercise early in the day.

- Reconsider naps that might make it difficult to sleep later.

- Keep your sleep environment cool, dark and quiet without TV or computer.

- Optimize your mattress and pillows.

- Relax through the evening—avoid stimulants like TV news or working.

- Maintain your nutrition plan.

- Keep your blood sugar steady and in your optimal zone.

- Remember you are your own best advocate and sleep serves you.

The influence of blue light deserves another mention. Our phones and computers and television sets and many light bulbs emit a wavelength of light that is designated blue even though we see it as white. Blue light detracts from your sleep prep because it blocks melatonin, the hormone that makes you sleepy. When you're not sleepy you postpone going to bed. Or you go to bed but not to sleep.

WebMD lists ways to manage our exposure to blue light:

- Cut back on screen time starting two-to-three hours before bed.

- Set an alarm for one hour before bed to quit using electronic devices.

- Dim the brightness on your devices.

- Install blue-light-filtering apps.

- Wear blue-light-blocking glasses.

- Swap light bulbs.

- Use a dim red lightbulb as a nightlight.

Lifestyle changes to enhance sleep are crucial. Both duration and quality of sleep affect our moods, our effectiveness and our blood sugar. When I get extra hours of sleep I wake humming and see a happy face in my bathroom mirror. When I wake after too-brief sleep, I am stiff muscled, bad-tempered, less effective at whatever I need to do that day, and exhausted by midafternoon. I haven't tracked my blood sugar levels as they align with satisfying sleep. But I suspect that when my blood sugar travels smoothly across the hours at 100 or so I have slept the best.

Clearly this is a quality of life issue! Lack of sleep affects us body, mind, heart and soul.

I found a quotation that expresses sleep's value for a man many of us admire.

Proper sleep has helped me get to where I am today as an athlete, and it is something that I continue to rely on every day.

Tom Brady
Quarterback with Seven Super Bowl Wins

A Few Extra Tips
Healthline.com published an article updated in February 2020 titled "17 Proven Tips to Sleep Better at Night." Some have already been covered, but here is an abbreviated list of their tips not yet listed.

- Increase bright light exposure during the day.

- Take a melatonin supplement.

- Consider other supplements including lavender and magnesium.

- Relax and clear your mind in the evening.

- Take a relaxing bath or shower.

- Don't drink any liquids before bed.

No one on my health care team has asked me about my sleep and I have not brought it up. I may not want to hear what medical experts advise. I fear another diagnosis and proposed treatment that adds to my daily list of must-dos. And yet… with proper treatment I might sleep better, feel better, live longer, yada, yada. I have not resolved my sleep issues. Even when it's 10 p.m. and I know I'm getting up early, I get a second wind and want to do things.

Sleep and its challenges bring up a topic we all face: how willing am I to do what is necessary for my good health? I have to decide whether shifting my lifestyle for better sleep is worth doing. With deep restful sleep I could dream better, my body could recover fully, and I could be better able to do all that I am called to do as a human being who happens to have type 1 diabetes. I just might have to struggle a little to get there.

It is also vital to address my sleep habits because there may be further complexities.

In February 2020, *Nature and Science of Sleep* published the article, "Sleep-related disorders in patients with type 1 diabetes mellitus: current insights." The article reported that researchers reviewed a number of studies and concluded that, "The prevalence of sleep problems appears to be higher among individuals with T1DM."

Examples of sleep problems follow.

Sleep Apnea

People with sleep apnea stop and start breathing while asleep. Their bodies partly wake them up to breathe. Apnea interferes with deep sleep and is associated with excessive snoring, nighttime wakefulness, morning headaches, bad moods, high blood pressure and daytime drowsiness. It also may eliminate dreaming and result in any number of personal difficulties, including relationship upheaval.

When faced with regular fatigue, feeling depressed, and uncontrolled blood sugar despite a healthy lifestyle, consider sleep apnea. Find out from your medical team how likely you are to have apnea. If your primary care physician thinks you do have apnea, he or she will usually recommend a sleep study.

Should your sleep study result in an apnea diagnosis, there are numerous techniques to try for sleeping better.

A study reported in the *American Journal of Respiratory and Critical Care Medicine* gives these directions for addressing obstructive sleep apnea:

- Exercise your tongue and throat. For example, repeatedly slide the tip of your tongue along your soft palate from front to back. Or five times a day place the tip of your tongue between your teeth and swallow five times.

- Stop sleeping on your back.

- Elevate the head of the bed so you do not sleep flat.

- Lose weight.

- Never drink alcohol at night or take drugs that relax your muscles.

- Stop smoking.

If apnea is severe and those changes are not enough, your medical provider may recommend a continuous positive airway pressure (CPAP) machine and mask. One online pundit reported that once diagnosed, sleep apnea can be *easily* treated with machines that force oxygen into your air passages. *Easily?* I doubt that he or his sleeping partner have apnea.

When I traveled with my sister and we shared a hotel room she told me I snored. Since *excessive* snoring is one sign of sleep apnea, I have wondered. Ideally I don't have sleep apnea and neither do you. But whatever sleep dysfunction you or I might be diagnosed with, and whatever extra care is prescribed, the resulting excellent sleep would nurture us on every level. Once more in my tango, I may have to master a new step.

Restless Leg Syndrome

Restless leg syndrome is also considered a common complication for people with type 1 diabetes. This syndrome produces creeping, crawling, tingling or painful sensations in the legs while you are trying to sleep. Experts have not developed a diagnostic test for restless leg syndrome, but link it with high blood glucose, thyroid disorders, or kidney problems. As with so many other complications, we may not know the actual cause. But iron deficiency, caffeine, and smoking may have an effect. Massage, stretches, either hot or cold compresses, and prescription drugs might bring relief.

Night Seizures

Severe hypoglycemia can cause seizures, so controlling hypoglycemia is the best approach for stopping seizures. Insulin pumps and CGM alarms can warn us of hypo or stop our insulin uptake. Spouses may rouse us when hypo has us restless and tossing in bed. And trained diabetes service dogs may sense hypo and wake us. I had a Siamese cat years ago who woke me from hypoglycemia. I never knew how she recognized my low blood sugar or how she determined that I needed to be awakened. But she relentlessly walked on me and talked to me until I got up, checked my blood sugar, confirmed that I was low and drank juice to come back to normal.

Insomnia

Insomnia.net points out that insomnia occurs most broadly in elders and those with obesity. And they add other reasons for sleeplessness that probably affect all of us and all sleep troubles.

- Depression

- Beliefs

- Social changes

- Hormonal changes

- Medication

- Pain and other discomfort

Reading that list I think of other aspects of T1D life that may disrupt sleep. Lack of safety concerns me. Feeling unsafe stands in the way of good sleep and I have not seen that listed anywhere in my research. It is not hard to imagine the uneasy sleep of people in a dangerous area or dangerous situation.

Worry is another potential sleep disturber. Any of us is prone to worry when contemplating health challenges or job loss or relationship drama or any life challenge. All of us are at risk in one way or another. I remember driving the interstate through the West years ago and looking off into canyons, thinking that humans have been in danger for all of time. Aboriginal people living in those canyons must have feared too much or too little rain, childbirth, not enough food, tribal censure, and attacks by predators of all kinds. It seems to be part of human nature to have to deal with known and unknown dangers. Perhaps earlier people were less likely to worry. But I worry and I know that many of us worry. And it affects our sleep.

Sleep is life and reflects our challenges. When nothing seems to be working to help us sleep, some experts recommend meditation and relaxation techniques or therapy. Sleep therapy may include lifestyle modifications, relaxation training and psychological or cognitive behavioral treatments. That makes perfect sense. When your days lead to sleepless nights, you cannot rest and recover. If your sleep does not support you, know that you are resourceful and can make changes that benefit your sleep, your diabetes and your life. If you have no remedies for poor sleep or sleeplessness, remember that we are not alone on the planet. Ask for help.

When I am sleepless, my mind follows an endless worry path about family, work, my inadequacies, what I have done and what I haven't done. How might I let that go? Breathing deeply and fully is my main approach. As I concentrate on sending my breath up and down the center of my body, connecting me with heaven and earth, I stop thinking and fall asleep.

As a person partnering with type 1 diabetes, I continue to perfect my health tango, adding beneficial regenerating sleep to my foundation.

By helping us keep the world in perspective, sleep gives us a chance to refocus on the essence of who we are. And in that place of connection, it is easier for the fears and concerns of the world to drop away.

Ariana Huffington
Author & Co-Founder of the *Huffington Post*

PART 5

AS THE DIS-EASE TURNS WHAT CAN YOU DO?

CHAPTER 16

Complications Great & Small

It may be a long stretch, but writing this chapter made me think of the plagues that the book of Exodus says God imposed on Egypt when the Pharaoh would not let the Israelites leave. At times the complications of type 1 diabetes seem like those biblical disasters. But are T1D disasters inevitable? No! The most important thing to know about complications of type 1 diabetes is that they are not inevitable. I repeat, complications are *not* inevitable.

And I warn you that this particular chapter is medically dense.

Harvard University's Joslin Diabetes Center in 2011 published results from the ongoing Medalist Study with 350+ people who had lived with type 1 diabetes for more than 50 years. Study results indicated that a high proportion of the Medalists remained free of complications (specifically retinopathy, kidney disease, neuropathy and cardiovascular disease). Researchers found it wasn't all about good blood sugar either—there were a number of other factors at play. But they ended the description of their research like an old joke, "Unfortunately we don't know what they are!"

Despite further investigation, researchers still have not identified those protective factors. In 2017, Joslin published further information on the Medalists. Researchers determined that, "Better management is linked to lower risks of cardiovascular disease, the leading cause of death in this population." Better management included blood glucose control and exercise. Beliefs and attitudes were not considered.

Beliefs and attitudes are powerful. Diabetic foot ulcers, for example, were addressed in a 2014 study on illness beliefs authored by the International Diabetes Federation. Researchers concluded that "Patients' beliefs [plus their understanding and their perception of their own control] are important determinants of foot-care practices. They may, therefore, also be influential in determining ulcer outcomes."

Keeping the ABCs in the recommended range is our best protection on a physical level. Poor control of the ABCs—average blood sugar, blood pressure and cholesterol—makes us more susceptible to physical trouble and means we either heal more slowly or maybe don't heal.

And of course there is a world of possibility beyond the physical. Along with beliefs, attitude is essential. If diabetes is a burden, then you struggle to bear it. If diabetes is a curse, then you are cursed. If diabetes is an enemy, you must go to war. Instead you might choose to designate diabetes as your ally.

Partnering with diabetes is my choice. I allow myself to feel all of the emotions that come up about my diabetes and its effects. Then

I spend most of my time with emotions that serve me, and take steps to recover from the rest. Deep compassion and love for myself help me stay healthy and happy. With love and compassion I can allow myself grief and sorrow and rage and all the spectrum of my feelings without getting highjacked.

Unfortunately, even good attitude and *perfect control* don't always work. For better or worse, although you may do everything right, things can go wrong. That's true in life and in diabetes. There are so many factors that affect your health and happiness.

Some people with type 1 diabetes have incurred no complications, and others have contracted terrible consequences—whether from BG difficulties, neglect, or bad advice and treatment. Although it is said that we can control type 1 diabetes, not everything can be controlled. If you or someone you care about have experienced extreme complications please accept my deep empathy for you.

Along with a positive attitude we best serve our bodies by keeping our blood sugar near normal. One of the concepts I stress with clients is that diabetes doesn't harm us. High blood sugar harms. Besides potentially causing immediate jeopardy, high blood sugar works over time to manifest further difficulties.

Sometimes, no matter how hard we try, our diabetes is uncontrolled. I experienced that over my early years when less was known about diabetes and I was surviving on a single daily injection of NPH with no access to my blood sugar levels or methods to cover carbs or treat highs. I did develop eye challenges.

All people with type 1 or type 2 diabetes are considered at risk for blindness and kidney disease. The small blood vessels in our eyes and kidneys are particularly susceptible to trouble from high blood sugar. I have told school kids that high sugar thickens the blood and causes harm as it flows through the body. "Does our blood turn into ketchup?" one student demanded. You could say that. Thickened blood, like ketchup, damages the small tender vessels in our eyes and kidneys.

Minor Sidetrack about Kidney Health

Although this book is not a comprehensive healthcare tome, I was advised to provide further information about kidney disease. The reason was reported in a 2019 article in the journal *Diabetes Care*, "Risk Factors for Kidney Disease in Type 1 Diabetes." The article's introduction states, "The lifetime risk of kidney disease in type 1 diabetes (T1D) has traditionally been estimated at ~50% but may exceed 70%."

With T1D we are 70% more likely to get kidney disease! Hearing that daunting assessment, it is helpful to know that there are five stages of chronic kidney disease and we do not all advance to kidney failure. Aging alone usually puts us in stage 1. Once you discover which stage you are in, with certain risk factors optimized, you can stabilize and perhaps even improve your kidney health.

That study's results came from observations of the Diabetes Control and Complications Trial (DCCT) cohort over an average of 27 years. A number of risk factors were investigated, including blood pressure, cholesterol, age, family history, medication use and presence of other complications. Researchers determined that "higher mean glycemic exposure was the strongest determinant of kidney disease among the modifiable risk factors." Once more we are reminded that keeping our blood sugar in the recommended range counts!

The National Kidney Foundation (NKF) reveals that kidney disease may develop slowly with few symptoms. And the *Diabetes Care* article further states that indicators of reduced kidney function may be unpredictable for type 1s. Knowing what leads to kidney trouble is vital.

Ten symptoms of kidney trouble are listed on the NKF website—kidney.org. They are:

1. tired, less energy, trouble concentrating
2. trouble sleeping
3. dry and itchy skin
4. need to urinate more often
5. blood in your urine
6. foamy urine
7. persistent puffiness around your eyes
8. swollen ankles and feet
9. poor appetite
10. cramping muscles

The NKF urges all Americans at high risk or over age 60 to get their kidneys checked annually. They also recommend that medical providers regularly check for kidney disease risk factors and help us control what we can control. It is wise for those of us with T1D to know the signs and remind our medical team members to check our kidneys and help us improve. If you have several of these symptoms, see your medical provider immediately.

The NKF lists items you might look for on your lab results and ask your doc about. The most important terms they mention are:

- Estimated GFR—glomerular filtration rate—tells how well your kidneys filter your blood.

- Albumin to Creatinine Ratio—estimates the amount of protein in your urine.

We are not alone. The NKF notes that one in three U.S. adults are at risk for kidney disease. Kidney disease is reported to kill more people than breast or prostate cancer! I didn't know that. Did you?

—

Our blood sugar control counts now and in the future. The terms *metabolic memory* or *legacy effect* describe the discovery that either poor or optimal blood sugar control over several years affects the likelihood of complications. Our bodies remember and react to what we have done in the past.

Good care now lasts. We are at our best and most likely to remain well when we maintain blood sugar in the recommended range. Current technology is exceedingly helpful and a competent medical team is essential. With those aids and a positive attitude you are most likely to stay well.

With my own susceptibility in mind, I closely watch and listen when people who have endured terrible complications of diabetes describe their life changes and how they dealt with them. Often they credit their losses with positive results—including different but greater self-awareness and ability. Even what seems like the worst can be incorporated in a favorable way.

Looking for goodness to report about vision loss I found Canadian artist Suzanne Gardner in an internet search. Despite laser treatments and surgery, retinopathy rendered her legally blind after years of type 1. Since then she has become a renowned painter. In a 2016 interview posted on Diabetes.co.uk Gardner said, "I really only learned how to appreciate the brilliance of the colours after my vision was almost gone."

Kidney failure is another terrible complication of diabetes and calls for either dialysis or a kidney transplant. Both are complex. Good news? A kidney transplant from a deceased donor may even include a pancreas—which makes the recipient non-diabetic for at least a while. At a writing workshop in Yellowstone National Park, I met a T1D in her fifth year without insulin injections after a kidney/pancreas transplant.

For most of us, vision loss or kidney disease can be postponed or halted by maintaining good blood sugar and blood pressure control. But even thinking about complications may bring up fear, sorrow, anger or hopelessness. When faced with something as challenging and uncertain as type 1 diabetes, it's natural to step into fear.

We know what to do to physically address complications. But how do we address our feelings about them? Despite the power of positive thinking, loss of any physical functioning is difficult.

Your complications may be devastating at times. The ongoing trouble with my eyes has been devastating for me. At about 20 years with T1D I discovered retinopathy and drifted into glaucoma, early cataracts and macular edema. Each has precipitated further treatment, some vision loss and greater self-awareness.

How do I get un-devastated? I do all that I can to maintain my ABCs. And I *believe* that I can stay well. Although I express my frustrations, I stay as positive as possible. I realize daily how productive and satisfying my life is, and I notice and stay grateful for what *is* working. I add specialists to my medical team and embrace the latest approaches for managing my imbalances. I keep my inner and outer eyes on beauty in my life and my world. And I love and appreciate myself, exactly as I am.

Nothing is inevitable. If we get complications, also known as comorbidities (and what an ugly word that is), those conditions have a good chance of being stabilized, improved or healed. Uncontrolled blood sugar is the usual culprit you can address. If your blood sugar is not in goal range, or you are having trouble staying in that range, meet with your medical provider or your diabetes educator for information, medication adjustments and encouragement. Don't put it off.

If complications have entered your life, adjust your team to include the very best medical experts for those complications. Again, don't wait.

And consider employing alternative aid. Find a provider who knows about acupuncture for your particular condition, or herbs and vitamins or special exercises or breathing techniques. Once I filled two pages with a handwritten list of all the alternatives I have tried over my years with type 1. Right now I take several supplements for my eyes, kidneys, circulation and other special needs. I read books and take courses on comprehensive approaches to healing. I keep track of inspirational speakers and writers and return to their works during down times. They lift my spirits and remind me that I can choose how I respond to challenges. The internet has numerous informational and heartening websites and blogs for people with type 1 diabetes. Connect with your T1D neighborhood.

It's also crucial for your good health to love, admire and educate yourself. Become the healthiest happiest human you can imagine being. Find a counselor, a coach or a spiritual advisor and stay in touch. Build optimism and joy into your life. Get involved with physical activity that you like doing. Create an exciting food plan and love what you eat. Spend time with people who appreciate you. Do work that satisfies you. Find your very own approach to living fully. Enrich your life and know how much you matter.

Meanwhile, for several reasons it might be helpful for you to know about the possible complications of type 1. This knowledge can help you think about your future. Like planning for retirement, you can take healthy steps now to assure that you stay well throughout your life. If you are fearful, use fear as a motivator so you do everything you can to avoid potential pitfalls.

What you are about to learn is simply information to help you stave off trouble. When you consider the following list of possible complications, be grateful for any that have not emerged, and know that the ones you have are manageable. I still occasionally fear losing my sight, but I see well enough for how I live. Every day I am thankful that my retinopathy is stabilized, that I am in good blood sugar control, and that I have strong legs and can walk.

Whenever possible, celebrate your good control. The Behavioral Diabetes Institute in San Diego sells a mug with this inscription—*News Flash: Well-Managed Diabetes is the Leading Cause of...*

Nothing! Well-managed diabetes is the cause of nothing. I like that thought. But if I'm in good control, can I get complications anyway? I was smacked with the idea of inescapable complications when I met my first endocrinologist. She came to my town once a week from a city 65 miles away and it was considered a coup to be able to see her. I had turned 30, had no complications, and wanted to learn more about my diabetes. The touted endocrinologist borrowed an office in a local clinic. I recall that it was a cold dark room with no windows. Darkness is a fitting memory since she felt it was her duty to warn me that my life with diabetes would only get worse. Bustling in, encased in a starched white coat, she checked my lab results. My liver, kidneys, cholesterol and thyroid looked good she said, "But of course things will go badly as you age." She reeled off every terrible consequence of diabetes that I could expect.

Whatever help that doctor offered me is lost. Her name is lost. I cannot picture her face. All I remember is the dark room and her insistence on all the suffering coming my way. She had no idea who I was or how I was taking care of myself. Her credo was, "Warn people with diabetes that they are doomed!"

As was my style then, I left without speaking up, sat in my car and sobbed. I was definitely scared of what diabetes might do to my body and my life. But I had always assumed that I would stay well, and I tried hard not to fall prey to the dire expectations of supposed experts. I certainly wasn't sure I could avoid complications, nor did I know how to prevent them. That's what I had hoped to learn from that specialist. It took days for me to recover from the negativity she dumped on me. I saw her once more to determine whether she might alter her approach for a second visit and teach me how to improve. She did not and I never returned.

In contrast, I recall visiting a hand specialist. The fingers on both my hands snapped closed and I had to manually pry them open. There were nodules on my finger joints. My hands ached, and their unnatural clutching distressed me. As a writer, a knitter, a seamstress, a cook and a gardener, I didn't want to lose function in my fingers and hands. I took my own advice and met with a specialist.

Most of this hand doctor's clients were dedicated athletes. He dressed like an athlete in comfortable clothes and running shoes. His exam room was bright and had windows looking into a beautiful garden. He walked across the room smiling and shook my hand, welcoming me.

Arms crossed and looking thoughtful, he concentrated as I listed my concerns. He told me the medical term for what I described was Dupuytren's contracture, and diabetes was one of its risk factors. (Web MD defines Dupuytren's contracture as an abnormal thickening and tightening of the normally elastic tissue beneath the skin of the palm and fingers. In severe cases, it can lead to crippling hand deformities.)

The doctor said Dupuytren's was not considered curable, but my symptoms could be alleviated. I asked what he meant by alleviated. He explained that treatment could help my achiness and soften the snapping sensation. Steroid injections were the primary nonsurgical treatment at that time, and if my symptoms greatly worsened, he could perform surgery. (There are more choices now.)

"What would you like to do?" he asked.

His manner made it possible for me to answer truthfully and with humor. Since I am perpetually dehydrated and was not interested in medical intervention I said, "I don't want steroid injections or surgery. I want you to tell me to drink more water."

"Then drink more water," he laughed.

We talked a little more. He suggested I massage my hands regularly. I agreed. When I suggested applying vitamin E oil to my hands he said, "Whatever makes you feel better is worth doing." We shook hands again and I left feeling cheerful. I worked on my blood sugar and massaged my hands with vitamin E oil, got some acupuncture, and over time my fingers actually healed. They don't contract or clutch. The nodules have dissolved. My hands are agile and serve me well.

When I saw those two specialists, not so much was known about the long-term consequences of type 1 diabetes. The Diabetes Control & Complications Trial (1982-1993) had not yet shown the value of tight blood sugar control. But meeting with the pleasant supportive doctor who listened to me reinforced my positive attitude about my future with diabetes. His attitude was uplifting and he reminded me that my health was literally in my hands.

You may benefit from knowing what's considered factual when learning about complications. Then when a not-so-positive specialist advises you, you have more information to help you find your own way. Be inquisitive. Select helpful advisors. Consider taking a wellness workshop or finding a type 1 peer to exchange information with. Search the internet for diabetes bloggers with experiences like yours.

It is valuable for you to know exactly where you stand on the diabetes health spectrum. Then you can evaluate your self-care and monitor any changes. You can check your own blood pressure and blood glucose. But you need laboratory tests for other essentials, like cholesterol, kidney function and thyroid values, and to affirm your A1c. Meanwhile, some providers are replacing the A1c with the Glucose Management Indicator (GMI) recorded on a CGM—which you can access for yourself.

When you have blood drawn or urine tested at a lab, request that the results be sent to you as well as to your doc. I review them ahead of my appointment so I know where I stand and what to ask my doctor about. I keep all copies to track how I'm doing over time.

Read this chapter or anything about complications only when you feel strong and ready to learn, so you aren't overwhelmed. Or read it with a loved one by your side so you can discuss it with them or at least hold their hand.

Be extra nurturing as you consider your lab results, and as you read about complications. Some people keep a hand on their hearts. Some put a bubble of white light around their lab results or this chapter. Remember that your actions matter and nothing is inevitable.

Complications occur on many levels, including the physical, emotional and worldly. Worldly complications are not on the medical lists below but include cost, discrimination, and isolation.

Forbes published an article in November 2018 with the headline "This Is The Shocking Cost Of Type 1 Diabetes." Author Lela London opened the article with suitable drama.

> Type 1 diabetes is all consuming. The stigma of misinformation. The inescapable quest for medical perfection. The 65,000-plus injections per lifetime (a lifetime which tends to be slashed 12 years from average as soon as you're diagnosed).
>
> The autoimmune disease takes hold of young bodies and never lets go. Without reason. And with no warning of the ever-expanding costs.
>
> A day in the life of a diabetic is an uphill battle. One that requires constant cognisance of the individual's food intake,

energy output, blood sugar levels, general health, and equipment (glucose meters, needles, insulins, food) that keeps them alive.

She cites a type 1 who limited insulin because she couldn't afford it, and went into diabetic ketoacidosis, which resulted in a $100,000 hospital bill. She also mentions a survey by Dexcom (makers of continuous glucose monitors), where 76% of respondents claimed to be "suffering stress, anxiety attacks or bouts of deep depression." In addition, 52% of those Dexcom surveyed reported feelings of anguish and anger over regular blood glucose checks.

Take a breath.

Insulin, which is our lifeline, has often been in the national news because the cost has risen outrageously. Some reports indicate that one vial of insulin, which lasts 28-42 days, costs more than $1,000 without insurance. In May 2020, a deal was cut nationally so that Medicare recipients with specific drug plans in 2021 would have a maximum insulin copay of $35 a month. What about those not on Medicare? And what about Medicare clients who reach the donut hole faster because the insurance company still claims to be paying thousands as their share of your insulin cost? In 2021 my insulin copay rose from $105 for a 90-day supply to $522 in June—so the realistic cost lasted only half a year.

Blood glucose testing strips too have increased to a punitive price. It is clear that companies are making billions on these supplies that are essential for good diabetes care.

A Mayo Clinic report in January 2020 documented when type 1s not on a continuous glucose monitor might need to check their blood sugar. The report suggested:

- Before meals and snacks
- Before and after exercise
- Before bed
- During the night (sometimes)
- More often if you're ill
- More often if you change your daily routine
- More often if you start a new medication

Good God! Not only are we constantly sticking ourselves to draw blood, but we are spending life savings to support the CEOs of companies manufacturing blood glucose test strips. CGMs are discussed elsewhere, but even with a CGM you may need to use a meter and strips. My dietitian friend on a Medtronic CGM has to calibrate twice daily with finger sticks, strips and a meter. I have to calibrate occasionally when my CGM doesn't accept the code I enter or circumstances otherwise go wrong.

On a trip to Glacier National Park before switching to a CGM, I ran out of strips. I was testing my blood sugar often while hiking and sightseeing and had forgotten to bring an extra vial of strips with me. I called the nearest pharmacy and was quoted $85 for 50 strips that worked in my particular meter. My insurance company would not contribute because I had refilled my strips prescription before I left home. I bought a ReliOn meter and strips at Walmart for a reasonable price. (At my last check Walmart's cost for 100 ReliOn strips was $17.88.) Although reviews favor certain types of meters and strips, all must meet certain standards to be on the market.

In January 2019, the *New York Times* reported that, "The sticker price is the result of behind-the-scenes negotiations between the strips' manufacturer and insurers. Manufacturers set a high list price and then negotiate to become an insurer's preferred supplier by offering a hefty rebate."

"Test strips are basically printed, like in a printing press," wrote David Kliff, who publishes a newsletter on diabetes economics (diabeticinvestor.com). He estimated that the typical test strip costs *less than a dime* to make.

Costs for care of diabetes continue to multiply when we have ongoing complications. My bimonthly eye injections for diabetic macular edema 2018-2020 cost about $2,000. My longer-range injection of a low-level steroid capsule cost more than $10,000 and is supposed to last two years. But I will probably need shorter-range booster shots during that time frame. My insurance, which is not cheap, paid for those injections. Without insurance I could not have afforded the injections, and I might have lost my sight.

Emotional complications are fully documented in articles, journals, books and webinars on type 1 diabetes. The main three repeated are anxiety, stress and depression. Discrimination and isolation have been added because they occur more often than we realize. When U.S. Supreme Court Justice Sonia Sotomayor was being vetted for acceptance to that court, critics wondered aloud on national TV whether she could do that job with type 1 diabetes. She has now successfully fulfilled her duties since 2009.

Discrimination has probably affected all of us and may hurt most when focused on children. In my diabetes educator's waiting room one September, a child came in weeping. Her mother explained that her daughter's entire school class had been invited to a party, but her child was left out because the party giver "didn't know what to feed her."

The Official Lists

Beyond cost, discrimination and the actuality of dealing with day-to-day care, these are complications the medical world links with type 1 diabetes. Remember these are probably linked with high blood sugar, not diabetes. Above all, remember that complications are not inevitable.

Broadly Cited Complications of Type 1 Diabetes (High Blood Sugar!)

- Circulation loss

- Eye disease

- Foot problems (nerve damage, poor blood flow, calluses, ulcers, amputations, Charcot foot)

- Heart disease

- High blood pressure

- Kidney disease (nephropathy)

- Low thyroid

- Nerve disease (neuropathy)

- Skin infections

- Slow digestion

- Slow wound healing

- Stroke

- Urinary tract infections

- Yeast infections

Lesser Known Complications of Type 1 Diabetes (High Blood Sugar!)

- Accelerated aging

- Cataracts (early)

- Dehydration

- Dementia

- Dry or itchy skin

- Dupuytren's contracture

- Eating disorders

- Frozen shoulder

- Gastroparesis (slowed or stopped stomach muscle contractions that keep the stomach from emptying properly)

- Gum disease and tooth loss

- Hearing loss

- Liver disease

- Low testosterone and infertility in males

- Osteoporosis

- Pain

- Psychological disorders (distress, depression, anxiety)

- Sexual dysfunction

- Sleep disturbances (apnea, restless leg syndrome, seizures)

- Tendons, muscles or fascia shortened

Other complications you may have heard linked with diabetes, like psoriasis and Parkinson's disease, have been connected with type 2 diabetes but not type 1.

Wait, There's More

Some experts believe that because type 1 diabetes is an autoimmune disease, type 1s are more likely to have other autoimmune disorders. Genetics are blamed, but no one knows exactly why autoimmune diseases might coexist.

Celiac disease, for example, is said to be associated with type 1 diabetes because it occurs more frequently in us than in the general population, and this association may be present in reverse. Researchers worldwide suspect that celiac might even be a precursor to type 1 diabetes, so are looking into gluten fed to infants and whether that relates to developing type 1.

Autoimmune Conditions Thought to Be Associated with Type 1

- Addison's disease

- Autoimmune arthritis

- Autoimmune gastritis

- Celiac disease

- Lupus

- Multiple sclerosis

- Thyroid diseases including Graves' and Hashimoto's

- Vitiligo

Now that you have seen a list of dreadful possibilities, how will you keep them away? Your body is your vehicle for life on earth. Is it getting the fuel, the love and the overall care it needs?

There are as many approaches to living as there are people on earth.

With type 1 diabetes we will be more likely to stay well for a lifetime if we take excellent care of ourselves. Our ongoing self-care, our traumas and any complications can be addressed with lifestyle change and alternatives as well as traditional medical treatment. Call on your team members to advise, perhaps to treat, and always to understand and inspire. We all benefit from partnership with those who respect us and lift our spirits.

In 1986, before we were connected to the worldwide web, and also before many books on diabetes were published, I found tremendous solace in the book *Love, Medicine & Miracles*. One of the author's quotes has guided me for years, and the research supports it.

Pessimists are more often right about life. But optimists are happier, and they live longer.

Bernie Siegel
MD, Surgeon, Pediatrician, Author

CHAPTER 17

Sick Days

"It's just a sick day," I tell myself. "No big deal. I'll stay home."

Ideally, this *is* just a sick day, time to rest and renew. But when I don't feel well, there is often a whisper that a simple illness might quickly develop into a full-fledged emergency. My world, my family obligations, my work may urge me to ignore early symptoms and push on. But my ally type 1 demands that I pay close attention to my body's messages.

Here's an example: One morning you awake feeling not quite right. You know you should eat but you're not hungry and your stomach is queasy. You were blasted out of sleep at 3 a.m. when your CGM screeched that your blood sugar was dropping. You ate glucose tablets and couldn't get back to sleep. You'd like to ignore work but there's an important meeting today. You aren't sure whether you're really sick or simply tired. Maybe you're having a reaction to that spicy food you ate last night. You will probably feel better once you drink a cup of herb tea and get going. How do you decide what to do?

Medical advisors think it's a sick day if you clearly have an illness or infection. If you start feeling sick, they recommend you stay home (or if working at home, sign out). But *feeling sick* doesn't always mean you *are* sick. Before you decide whether you will push through and work, carefully track your bodily sensations. Check for headache, vision changes, sinus congestion, breathing problems, sore throat and so on all the way up, down and around your body. Determine whether anything unusual invites your attention. (I have nondiabetic friends who do this body check daily as part of their morning routine.)

Remember that stress plays a role. If you are going through a challenge in any part of your life, stress may affect your blood sugar and your health. Even more confusing, everyone's body handles stress differently. I attended a seminar led by two diabetes educators with type 1. Before their talk they stood on stage heads together adjusting their insulin pumps. One turned and explained that she was setting a temporary basal rate to keep the stress of presenting from raising her blood sugar. The other one laughed and told us she was doing the opposite—adjusting her basal rate to prevent stress from sending her too low!

Check your blood sugar. Is it too high, too low, in your goal range? Is your blood sugar steady or peaking and falling? Are you chasing and correcting unexplained highs? If you have a CGM, note trends. Is today's pattern different from most days?

Once you complete your full body check, stress assessment and blood sugar review, where do you stand? You may determine that you are just missing sleep and will revive, so you can work. Or you may admit that even though you aren't sick, you aren't feeling as good as you like to feel, and give yourself a day off. You might notice that your nose is running and you have a scratchy throat. That's my sign that I am catching cold and if I stop everything and rest now, I won't go all the way into it.

You might also discover that your body is sick, and you need to take time to recover. Promise yourself that you will listen to your body's warning system and do what's needed.

When You Decide that You Are Ill

Like it or not, solutions to most type 1 health upsets depend on you and your preparation. Whether you have a minor infection or the beginnings of a more serious dilemma, it is essential to recognize your body's signals, to have a good idea how to take care of yourself, and to have support. Your job is to get well, to stay well, and to avoid potential trauma. Fortunately, having type 1 diabetes can make you more aware overall, and can signal you when help is needed.

Any illness may take you into jeopardy and that is not a place you need to go. It's best not to hide or deny or ignore. Be prepared for a cold or the flu or a virus. Breathe deeply and gratefully and take action. Have food and juice and cough drops and cough syrup and insulin and blood glucose strips and ketone strips and over-the-counter meds to reduce fever and pain. And be prepared to call for help. Have your list of medical team members and their contact information handy.

It's an excellent idea to have a sick day plan and a sick day kit prepared. If you don't already have a plan, next time you visit your doctor or diabetes educator, ask for one you can personalize with their help. Once you have created your sick day plan, keep a printed copy readily available, even if you think you know it by heart. And have your medical team members in your phone contacts.

Sample Sick Day Plan

- Let a friend or family member know that you feel unwell so they can provide standby support.

- Check your blood sugar more often than usual. Is it low, high, steady or vacillating? (Many sick day plans advise checking blood sugar every two hours. When in doubt I check every half hour because things change fast and I want to know whether I'm improving or getting worse.)

- Doublecheck your CGM readings with a blood sugar meter before correcting for highs or treating lows. The CGM measures interstitial fluid rather than blood, so the numbers reported by the CGM are different. Checking blood sugar is especially important when your numbers are changing rapidly or dramatically.

- Be aware that your basal or carb coverage may need to change, possibly significantly. Know how to adjust your insulin and oral medications, if you need to.

- Check for ketones every 2-4 hours. Ketones may signal that your illness is worsening and you are headed for diabetic ketoacidosis. More information about DKA is provided in the True Emergencies chapter.

- Track continuing symptoms. If you think you are getting worse, call a member of your health team and run your symptoms, your blood sugar, and ketone results by them.

- Definitely call your doctor if you are vomiting or have diarrhea more than three times over 24 hours or have had a fever higher than 101° for 24 hours.

- Have easy and healthy foods and fluids available. Your appetite may increase or decrease, and if it does, be more careful than usual with insulin dosing.

- You will benefit from extra fluids, so keep drinking water. Have juice or sweetened sodas available in case you can't eat and your basal insulin takes you low.

Once you have a plan, come up with your sick day kit.

Sample Sick Day Kit
- A copy of your sick day action plan.

- A sliding scale for additional insulin doses or alternate basal/bolus rates provided by your MD or diabetes educator.

- Blood glucose meter and strips.

- Ways to measure ketones—urine testing strips or a meter with strips that can monitor blood ketones.

- Blood glucose diary or notebook and pen to keep track of your symptoms.

- Thermometer.

- Approved pain relief medication.

- Food and drinks for sick days, for example crackers, mineral water, oatmeal, soup.

- Drinks to keep you hydrated and keep your blood sugar steady if you can't eat, including regular soda, fruit juice.

- Hypo treatment (glucose tabs, juice, etc.) including glucagon—details in True Emergencies chapter.

- Insulin, pump and CGM essentials.

- Insulin syringes or pen to replace pump if needed.

Check your kit at least every six months to replace expired supplies, review phone numbers, and restock anything you have used. I put a reminder on my calendar.

Some over-the-counter medicines may send blood sugar levels high or low or interfere with readings on your glucose monitor or CGM. Talk about this with your diabetes educator or physician or call the company, so you can purchase pain relievers, cold remedies, cough medicine or cough drops that are right for you and have them ready in your sick day kit. Choose components you know work for you and that you like. For example, my coughs are best stopped by Ricola cough drops. I tried the sugar free drops and they gave me immediate diarrhea. I called the company and found out that the sugared drops have 3 carb grams each, so I take insulin to cover them.

If You Get Worse…

You have determined that you are ill, and your illness is not an emergency. However, it is still important to remember that with type 1 diabetes any ailment can become more serious. This chapter is all about encouraging you to stay on top of small issues so they don't blow up. If symptoms worsen or you are in doubt, call your doctor or educator. Your job is to get better, not worse. And on a day when you are well, review the True Emergencies chapter.

CHAPTER 18

True Emergencies
Out of Insulin, Environmental Disasters, Hypo, Hyper, DKA

At certain times type 1s are in deep trouble and may or may not know it. Threatening experiences include lack of insulin, ineffective insulin, environmental disasters, and severe hypoglycemia or hyperglycemia that you cannot recover from on your own.

No Insulin

The first type 1 emergency is to be without viable insulin. Being without insulin is a major vulnerability for a type 1. We must inject insulin at least daily or we head for death. For that reason, as well as many others we're exploring in this book, we type 1s must be brave and resourceful for our very survival.

Experiencing type 1 emergencies and handling them can build strength. The root of the word emergency is emergence—growth, transformation, evolution. My intention with this book is to help you benefit from every type 1 experience, and to inspire you to establish and maintain a healthy lifestyle and a healthy attitude. As you work to steady yourself and your diabetes, everything changes and changes again. Will you continue to evolve? Of course, you will!

Limited access to insulin is a terrible truth about having type 1. Insulin prices go up. Insurance companies establish ever-changing limitations. And the financiers deciding who gets how much insulin when, don't appreciate that you will die without it. Getting and having enough insulin is an ongoing challenge.

Expense is the primary reason that insulin might be limited or unavailable. The price of insulin has skyrocketed in recent years. On pre-pandemic television news I saw lines of U.S. type 1s getting on buses to go to Canada to buy reasonably-priced insulin. And I have seen weeping mothers recount their sons' and daughters' deaths because they tried to survive on limited insulin. In poorer parts of the world type 1s simply die because insulin is not available. International efforts to make insulin accessible to all are proceeding slowly. (Among others, the American Diabetes Association and beyondtype1.org list resources for access to insulin in the U.S.)

I saw a horrifying episode on a 2020 television medical drama where a boy was admitted to ER with high blood sugar and his mother was accused of not giving him insulin. She insisted that she gave him a shot every morning. Investigation revealed that she bought *insulin* on the black market because she couldn't afford what pharmacies charge. And the vial she bought was filled with water.

Insulin comes in many types and strengths and is patented and said to be complicated to produce. The term generic is controversial. But a Walmart pharmacist in 2021 informed me that ReliOn's Novolin N, R or 70/30 were available without prescription for about $25. You may know that those types of insulin are not the most recent, probably not recommended by your MD, and may not serve type 1 needs.

Better news for types 1s—as of mid-2021, Walmart and Sam's Club pharmacies carry a more-reasonably-priced ReliOn version of Novolog rapid-acting insulin. My local Walmart pharmacy told me they had ReliOn Novolog available without a prescription for $72.88 for a vial and $85.88 for a pen.

Even when you have insulin, it may not work.

Temperature Control

A vial or a pen filled with insulin is meant to be kept refrigerated until it's opened. Once in use it is meant to be kept at room temperature—defined by the U.S. Food & Drug Administration as 59° F to 86° F.

Your insulin *will* deteriorate if it freezes or cooks. It loses its effectiveness if stored in the glove compartment of your vehicle, left unprotected on the beach, or forgotten in your jacket pocket in the unheated coat room during a freeze. Once again, your safety is in your own hands. It is up to you to protect this precious stuff.

Literature enclosed in packages with insulin pens makes room temperature mandatory for a pen in use. How about vials? The tiny-print paperwork folded inside every insulin package affirms that there's a choice. For glargine (Lantus) insulin, for example,

Full Prescribing Information states that—unopened Lantus vials should be stored in the refrigerator until the expiration date; *in-use Lantus vials may be refrigerated or kept at room temperature protected from heat and light*. (http://products.sanofi.us/lantus/lantus.html#section-16.2)

It infuriates me that people with diabetes are told their insulin *must* be refrigerated while in use. I have confronted pharmacists and MDs who tell patients that, and they insist that people with diabetes can't be trusted to keep their insulin out of heat or cold or light. Keeping your insulin at a safe temperature and out of direct light does take attention and commitment but this is not rocket science! Numerous kits made to protect insulin are sold for those of us who transport it. I keep my backup vial in a *Frio* case that goes everywhere with me in my day bag. The *Frio* lining is filled with beads that absorb water. Evaporation keeps my insulin cool. I simply soak the lining when it dries—about every two days. No ice needed.

Not having to depend on refrigeration liberates you. Our bodies prefer insulin injected at body temperature. And type 1s on insulin need to have it with them.

Megan kept it in her insulated diabetes travel case when she toured Mexico. As a backpacker I wrapped my insulin in my sweater and stuffed it deep in my pack. My dad's friend Paul met him for breakfast at McDonald's with his insulin pen in his shirt pocket. Grandma Margaret keeps her basal insulin in the drawer beside her bed ready for her nighttime injection. We are humans with busy lives and need no meaningless barriers.

Insulin Beyond Its Use Date

Opened insulin has a use date. If your vial or pen has been in use for longer than the manufacturer advises it may not work at all, or it may work poorly. Insulin manufacturers say vials of the long-acting insulin detemir (Levemir) last 42 days after opening, and glargine (Lantus) vials last 28 days. Vials of the fast-acting insulins— aspart (Novolog) and lispro (Humalog) are said to last 28 days. Insulin pens vary in length of efficacy from 10-42 days. Know how long *your* insulin lasts.

To keep track of insulin's effectiveness, docs and pharmacists I have worked with recommend inking the date you *open* insulin on your vial or pen. But I think it's smarter to label your insulin pen or vial with the day it loses its effectiveness! Seeing that date every day reminds you to get ready to change to a fresh insulin source and trash the one you've been using.

Expired Insulin

Even when properly stored, unopened insulin expires—usually at least a year after you purchase it. Expiration dates appear on the vial or the pen or the box they come in. I was told years ago that insulin manufacturers had been directed to create long-lasting insulin that did not need refrigeration. For many reasons that has not been done. I suspect that having it expire is a financial guarantee. Insulin-making companies can count on steady revenue because we must have insulin and if it expires before it's used, too bad!

You may not realize that your insulin has lost its effectiveness until you inject it and your blood sugar doesn't respond. As a type 1, you will quickly realize that your insulin isn't effective. But I have worked with type 2s on insulin who didn't grasp that the insulin they used off and on for months wasn't working.

An elderly type 2 client of mine struggled to accept that insulin could *spoil*. Mr. Sanderson had been raised dirt poor and could not bear to waste. If there was insulin left in the vial, he used it. Even when he opened a new vial, he kept the old one *just in case*. His doctor put him on a CGM that revealed high blood sugar when he used the expired insulin. With that evidence, Mr. Sanderson finally began discarding his out-of-date insulin and opening a new vial when it was time.

If you find it necessary to use insulin beyond its recommended expiration date, keep checking your blood sugar to make sure that insulin is working.

Environmental Disasters

Whenever I hear about a natural disaster I wonder, "Are the type 1s going to make it?" That's not because we are more vulnerable to harm. It's because without insulin we're dead whether injured, homeless or not. When I listen to news reports about tropical storms devastating Caribbean Islands, or fires, tornadoes, landslides, blizzards, power outages and floods destroying homes in my own country, I pray.

If I were at work and couldn't get home to gather supplies, I do not have enough insulin to last long. I regularly carry my glucose monitor and one partly-filled insulin vial with two or three syringes, in case my pump stops working or I accidentally rip off my infusion set. But if I were banished without getting home, my pump would need to be charged, I would have no replacement infusion sets, no CGM accoutrements and my insulin supply would soon be depleted.

Manufacturers tell us to keep unopened insulin refrigerated to preserve it, so I don't take extra insulin with me on daily outings. And health insurance plans limit how much insulin we are given. How might any of us arrange to have enough insulin with us at all times to last for days or even weeks?

I imagine myself standing in line with hundreds of others after a disaster, convincing whoever's in charge that I have type 1 diabetes, and that I must have insulin. Off my pump I'd need two vials or two pens—one for basal insulin and one for bolus. It doesn't seem likely that the emergency medical unit thrown together on the rodeo grounds or a football field will have enough insulin to hand me two precious vials or pens.

As a human being on an ever-changing planet, you could abruptly be forced by outside forces into emergency mode. You could be facing a pandemic, out of work and even homeless. You could be wading through waist-high flood water. You could be clearing out of your home in 15 minutes to evade a raging fire. As a type 1, you are always at greater risk from these events.

Are you prepared to run for your life and cover your diabetes needs? I wonder how quickly I could gather essential documents, corral two housecats, find my hidden cash and maneuver all my diabetes gear into my car. Scattered all over my house are my pump and CGM supplies, vials of insulin that need to be kept cold, prescriptions, extra strips for my blood glucose monitor, clean clothes, cat food, etc., etc. My most important consideration must be: *Do I have insulin?*

If you live in an area where your home might be destroyed or you might be unable to return to it, it is vital that you have immediate access to whatever lets you maintain your type 1 health regimen.

Any of us might benefit from creating an emergency kit. Although I would still need to get home to pick it up, I now keep my insulin and syringes in the refrigerator in a soft-sided insulated lunchbox with a handle. The lunchbox would be easy to grab and would keep the insulin cool or safe from freezing. A month's pump and CGM gear are stashed in a cardboard box in a cupboard nearby. All I have to remember is to use and replace those components regularly so they don't expire.

My awareness about being prepared increased years ago when I joined a volunteer group giving out diabetes information at the state capitol during the legislative session. One of the volunteers was an undocumented Guatemalan community health representative who wore a fanny pack with all his diabetes gear in it. Brave and practical, he was prepared to take care of his type 1 needs even if he was arrested or deported. I swallow hard to keep tears away just remembering him.

Severe Hypoglycemia or Hyperglycemia

Type 1 emergencies always center around blood sugar, and we live with vacillating blood sugar daily. You are at risk if your blood sugar drops too low, and you are at risk if your blood sugar stays high.

If you are hypoglycemic and cannot take care of yourself and no one around you knows what to do, you have an emergency. When you have high blood sugar and cannot bring it down, you have an emergency. As always, check your blood sugar when in doubt and treat your lows or your highs. But even when you do everything you need to do you may still have trouble.

When your blood sugar is dramatically low or high, and you can't bring it back to normal, get help. Tell whomever you are with what you need. Or simply say, "Take me to an emergency room." For those who live alone, you might ask an acquaintance or even a stranger to contact your doctor, or 911, or transport you to an emergency room. Make it clear that you are not able to care for yourself—and tell them what you need. Most people will gladly help. They just need to know what to do for you.

Once while shopping in a big box store, I began to crash with hypoglycemia. I went to a checkout counter and told the cashier that I had diabetes and needed to drink something sweet. She helped me sit on a bench, brought me a coke, and kept an eye on me until I recovered. I am grateful that she knew enough NOT to call 911.

Another time I came close to needing help for high blood sugar after sharing brunch with new friends in a town 70 miles from mine. The hostess served Mimosas and delicious high-carb foods. I ate and drank too much. As a passenger sitting in the back seat on the way home, I kept checking my blood sugar and it wasn't coming down. I tried to explain to the person in the passenger seat that I might need to be taken to ER. She laughed at me and said, "You mean you overdid it!" I regretted not preparing my companions. And, thank God, as we continued toward home my blood sugar responded to the insulin I had taken and my emergency was averted.

As a type 1 you have to plan ahead, take action, stay with yourself no matter what's going on, and speak up. There will be events in your life when even the medical provider in charge has no idea what you need or how to save you. You may have to be the hero and rescue yourself. Be ready to be brave.

Hypoglycemia

Because we type 1s depend on unpredictable injected insulin, hypoglycemia can occur anytime without warning. Hypoglycemia is considered severe when a person's blood sugar drops so low that they need assistance to help them recover. Many of us have taken care of ourselves even at that level. I once lay on my living room floor with blood sugar at 20 mg/dL. No one else was around and I was too low to reach out, so I lay there and ate glucose tabs until I recovered.

The Mayo Clinic lists the following signs of low blood sugar:

- An irregular or fast heartbeat
- Fatigue
- Pale skin
- Shakiness
- Anxiety
- Sweating
- Hunger
- Irritability
- Tingling or numbness of the lips, tongue or cheek

As hypoglycemia worsens further symptoms may occur:

- Confusion, abnormal behavior such as the inability to complete routine tasks

- Visual disturbances, such as blurred vision

- Seizures

- Loss of consciousness

Your symptoms might be different. Or, because over the years many people with diabetes lose awareness of hypo symptoms, you might have no warning you can track. Your risk is greatly reduced if you know your signs or that you are unaware, and if you notify your friends, family and coworkers of your hypoglycemia behaviors before they are needed. They may already be aware that you change when your blood sugar drops. Friends I hike with tell me I get quiet and my eyes glaze over with hypoglycemia. They notice, stop, and make me eat or drink something sweet. They also know that recovery from hypoglycemia may take a while, so we all rest until I can check my blood sugar and see that I'm back in healthy range.

One of my clients was greatly relieved to hear that we express hypo in individual ways. Andrea had not realized that when she gets confused and aggressive, pushes family members away and can't complete a simple task, her blood sugar is low. She explained to her spouse and kids that those are signs she needs help. Now when Andrea behaves strangely her husband puts an arm around her and hands her an opened bottle of juice.

Low blood sugar affects the brain and thus your ability to act effectively. When I'm alone at home with hypo, I may stand for long moments with my refrigerator door open, unable to choose what to eat or drink to raise my blood sugar. I get hazy about what's best for me. Or I get stubborn and decide I don't want fruit or syrup or jam or any of the foods that might help me recover. My current remedy is to keep several small apple juice bottles on an easy-reach kitchen shelf. No decision needed. I just open a bottle and drink juice.

A type 1 friend of mine is a kind and warmhearted elementary school teacher. As a sign that lack of sugar is affecting her brain, Tanya gets bitchy. When she's in the classroom her low blood sugar personality change is obvious. Her students know where she keeps hard candy and they rush to make her eat it. Her low blood sugar could become an emergency and derail her day, but her students have been trained to step in and help her.

Without self-awareness or informed companions, your blood sugar may get so low that you are unable to eat or drink something sweet, or to communicate what's happening. The extreme reaction to hypo is unconsciousness, which is rare, but you need to be prepared.

Tanya shares a house with Jim, another type 1, and recently she found him lying on their kitchen floor unable to speak. He was committed to tight control and she knew he often had low blood sugar. She assumed that was the case and knew what to do. Jim was breathing well and able to swallow, so she left him lying on his side and carefully dribbled syrup into his mouth. Had he been unconscious, she knew that forcing food or drink into his mouth should never be done because he might choke. After administering the sweet syrup, she stayed beside him, phone in hand to call 911 if he didn't recover, and waited until he came back to full awareness, could sit up and eat or drink on his own.

Jim might confer with his endocrinologist and diabetes educator and adjust his insulin regimen to avoid extreme lows. He would benefit from a continuous glucose monitor to alert him of imminent lows. And he should have glucagon on hand and make sure his housemate knows how to use it. Wanting to keep your blood sugar within tight parameters is fine as long as you do it with the right tools and support.

There are also sweet gels available to put in your elderly mom's mouth when she can't chew. They are, of course, expensive, so my friend Martine keeps a tube of cake frosting beside her pillow at night that she can squeeze into her mouth if her blood sugar goes too low.

What about Glucagon?

The American Diabetes Association recommends that any of us who might ever have blood glucose lower than 54 mg/dL have glucagon available and teach people in our households how to apply it.

Glucagon is a hormone that stimulates the liver to release stored sugar and is the recommended remedy for severe hypoglycemia. It might be a life saver.

The original glucagon kits came with a powder and liquid that had to be combined and then injected by someone besides the person with hypoglycemia. Mixing and injecting were complex for those untrained, and T1Ds were discouraged from trying to do it ourselves. Therefore, individuals living alone have not thought it helpful. It was also expensive and expired quickly.

In 2019, glucagon was made longer-lasting and much easier to use. Choices now include a prefilled and ready-to-use syringe or pen for injections; or a powder to spray in the nose. Those kits last two years if unused. A co-worker, friend, family member or live-in companion can easily be trained to administer glucagon when you need it.

A glucagon injection or powder should bring the person quickly back, but medical experts advise following the glucagon with sweets as soon as the affected person can swallow, and calling for emergency help. While hypoglycemia might simply be caused by a mistake in insulin amounts or not eating, it might also be a sign of a more serious issue that needs to be medically addressed. Whether you follow glucagon with a call to ER or not, let your medical team know about such an episode.

Type 1s living alone might still reject the appropriateness of glucagon. But it is possible to administer it yourself. In 2020 I listened to two endocrinologists who are type 1s discuss injecting themselves with glucagon when their hypo was out of control. Their podcast, "Glucagon Saved Our Butts!" is worth watching, and available on Taking Care of Your Diabetes (tcoyd.org) or YouTube. They pointed out that both were experienced type 1s on insulin pumps and CGMs, but despite warnings were still vulnerable to extreme hypo. They advised that the new glucagon options are a valuable resource for any type 1.

Hyperglycemia

High blood sugar may also take type 1s into emergency status. Hyperglycemia often accompanies illness or stress and may lead to diabetic ketoacidosis (DKA). To explain DKA: even though you may be taking insulin, when it isn't working, sugar can't get into your cells. To compensate, the cells burn fat for energy. Your liver turns this fat into ketones and sends them into your bloodstream for muscles and other tissue to use as fuel. DKA happens when both glucose and ketones in the blood are too high. Ketone buildup dehydrates you, makes your blood too acidic, and robs your body of salts and fluids.

You can check for ketones with urine strips, a meter that checks for ketones in the blood, or a breathalyzer.

Signaling oncoming DKA, ketones spill into your urine, and ketone testing strips for urine are available at pharmacies without a prescription. You simply unwrap a strip, hold it in a stream of urine, watch for color change and compare results to the chart included with the strips. Urine ketone strips use the terms moderate or large for ketones that should be medically addressed. Moderate or large ketones are a sign of danger because they upset the chemical balance in your body.

A blood ketone meter is said to provide the most accurate results. Specific blood ketone meters are available, and certain blood sugar meters can test for ketones with special strips or a code.

Ketone breathalyzers measure acetone concentration in the breath and are not recommended.

The American Diabetes Association recommends checking urine for ketones every four to six hours when ill or when blood sugar is higher than 240 mg/dL. Without medical treatment DKA is life-threatening.

Signs of DKA include:

- High blood sugar that won't come down

- Ketones

- Nausea, vomiting, diarrhea

- Abdominal pain

- Rapid breathing or breathlessness

- Dry or flushed skin

- Drowsiness, inability to concentrate, confusion or weakness

- Increased thirst or dry mouth

- Frequent, reduced, or no urine output

- Breath that smells *fruity*

Call one of your medical team members and seek urgent medical attention if you have high blood sugar and any of these symptoms. Medical care is essential when blood glucose levels continue to rise even after you have taken at least two extra doses of insulin, are not well enough to follow your sick day plan or don't have anyone to help you.

You do *not* have to go all the way to DKA. There are signs along the way where you can intervene and steer yourself back to safety or enlist medical help. The last time I approached DKA, I was traveling when I had been only a week on an insulin pump for the first time. My own ignorance and bad choices built up to a real drama.

Travel prep is hell for me. As a former military brat, I still fear that once I leave home, I might never make it back. On the night before flying to South Carolina to see my dad, I fell into bed with only two hours to sleep, and never heard my alarm. My friend Patt woke me pounding on my bedroom window. It was too late for her to take me to the shuttle, so she left, and I lurched into action.

Throwing my suitcase and carry-on into my car I yelled goodbye to my cats and took off. It was 65 miles to the airport and I was late. My blood sugar surged upward as I accelerated down the dark highway. Once in the airport I stood panting in the security line. They rifled my carry-on looking for the wine corkscrew I had forgotten and hissed at me because I was hopping from foot to foot in anxiety. After a pat-down I made it past security and boarded my plane.

Once the plane took off and leveled out, I checked my blood sugar and it was in the 200s. I was starving and had left my carefully assembled breakfast at home. Knowing I should not (remember when your blood sugar is off, so might be your thinking), I ate the sweet snack the steward offered. My blood sugar went up. We landed in Atlanta a little late and my connection was tight, so I sprinted through the airport hearing the sound system paging me—the late passenger—to report to my boarding gate. I made that flight too. But my blood sugar went up. I checked every half hour and regularly took insulin to bring it down. My new pump didn't seem to be helping, so I started taking insulin by syringe.

Three time zones and hours after starting out, I met my dad at the Greenville, South Carolina airport. We went to a local café to drink iced tea. The waitress automatically served us southern-style sweet tea and I was parched so I drank it all. I checked my blood sugar for the 11th or 12th time and it was in the 400s. I was feeling the signs of ketoacidosis—exhausted, heavy legs, fast heartbeat, shallow breath.

"Dad," I said, "My blood sugar is really high and I think I'm in trouble."

He just looked at me.

"I'm going to call my diabetes educator," I said. Her clinic put me through to Paula and I told her what was happening.

"Have you checked your ketones?" she asked. I had not. In fact, I had never checked my ketones, so I didn't have test strips with me.

"Go to a pharmacy and get urine ketone strips. Call me back with your results," Paula commanded.

Dad drove me to a pharmacy. I bought the strips and went into the restroom to check. Once wet, my strip immediately darkened, showing moderate ketones. I called Paula and reported.

"Go to an emergency room now," she ordered.

We advanced to the hospital in my father's small town. The person who came downstairs to greet us in the empty emergency room slowly checked all my identification and confirmed that I was insured. She disappeared.

Collapsing onto a slick plastic chair I waited and was finally approached by a man in a lab coat followed by another man in scrubs.

"I am a doctor," the lab coat said, "Why are you here?" I explained how my day had gone, assured him that I had regularly taken extra insulin and still my blood sugar wasn't coming down.

He ushered me into an exam room and said, "I want to see you take insulin." I pulled 10 units of insulin into a syringe, bared my belly and injected it. He started to leave me alone to wait for the insulin to take effect.

But I said, "Look, I have type 1 diabetes and signs are that I am going into a coma with ketoacidosis. I need intravenous fluids and electrolytes."

He glared at me. I pulled out a ketone strip and held it up for him to see.

"I am going to pee on this strip," I said, "and I will show you that I have significant ketones."

When I came back with my darkened strip, he remained belligerent. But the man in scrubs was a nurse and knew more about my dilemma than the doc. He whispered to Dr. Don't-Believe-You and pulled him out of the room. When they returned, the doctor had apparently read the manual that tells how to treat ketoacidosis. Still judgmental, he ordered the appropriate treatment. The nurse attached the IV fluid and I sank back on the exam table, finally believing that I would be all right.

As far as support went, I knew my dad loved me but this situation was beyond his emotional capability. He had stayed in the waiting room ruffling through magazines while I was examined. As I was gratefully rehydrating, he came to find me.

"I'll be back," he said and went home to eat a sandwich. Having been raised to take care of myself, and knowing that when dad was overwhelmed he disappeared, I was disappointed but not surprised. He came back an hour later and I was released from ER, tired but recovered, with my blood sugar back in range.

I strongly remember that emergency experience for many reasons. My diabetes educator and the ER nurse saved my life. My father and the unwise doctor might have unwittingly let me die. In crucial moments, even near coma, I spoke up for myself. I am proud that I knew what to say and was able to convince the unenlightened doctor in charge.

Trained to be stoic, I don't ordinarily get emotional during such events. I know that type 1s need to be ever prepared to advocate for ourselves. Even in a hospital emergency room in the supposed care of an MD, I was the one who knew what to do. What if I had not spoken up? What if the more-knowledgeable nurse hadn't been there to convince the ER doc? What if I had no insurance card and the front door guard hadn't even let me in? What if my diabetes educator hadn't been available? Like scouts, we have to be prepared.

Yet I thought I was prepared and my trip would go smoothly. Having a new pump seemed like an asset. I didn't realize how much I didn't know. My diabetes educator thought I was used to depending on the backup of long-acting insulin—which was no longer there with a pump. But when problems showed up, I applied my resources. I knew I was in trouble. I did not ignore my symptoms. I kept trying things. I called a team member I trusted and could reach. I was willing and able to keep explaining and convincing even when I was headed for coma. I did not give up. I came through my emergency successfully and I gained courage for the future. I also called my primary care physician the next day and told her my story. She was both inquisitive and supportive, congratulating me for a successful completion to my emergency and thanking me for reporting in.

Type 1 diabetes adventures keep coming. This story reminds me that although my diabetes is *in control* and did not seem more demanding during the pandemic, I feared being hospitalized. Not only might Covid-19 kill me, but so could standardized care for a type 1 inpatient. How might overwrought RNs in a crowded hospital respond properly to my complex needs? (Carry a letter from your endocrinologist and stay in touch with a health care advocate.)

Instead of being on safari or skydiving or crossing the Pacific in a tiny sailboat (although you can do those things too), you must apply your knowledge and skills to diabetes experiences that can easily become life or death. You don't have to seek thrills; they are built into your condition. Type 1 is never boring. As Roseanne Roseannadanna repeated on Saturday Night Live, "It's always something."

In that small-town ER I moved past any hesitation and stepped into the situation calm and confident. Applying my expertise, I brought a possible tragedy to healthy completion. In full expression of the root meaning of emergency, I grew, transformed, evolved.

CHAPTER 19

Near-Death Experience

Looking closely at the potential danger of hypo, hyper, lack of insulin, etc., brings another issue into the light.

One looming aspect of type 1 diabetes is usually hidden, even from ourselves—we live near death. It's not a bad neighborhood. We can practice urban renewal and make everything more beautiful and precious. But it's essential to be protective of yourself when you live here and to find a way to go beyond.

In essence, every human lives near death, but most don't know it.

Knowing we live near death may take us to great heights or to ponderous depths, most likely both at different times. I got very mindful as a result of my diabetes diagnosis and dodged my feelings. Although I don't experience chronic pain, I learned to distance myself from the pain of finger sticks and injections. Consequently, I checked out of my feelings and my body. I have had to learn how to accept my emotions and recognize what body sensations are telling me.

"Put your hand on your heart when you leave your body," my counselor Annette coached me as a recent session ended, "and come home." That was a new idea and a new sensation. I haven't been home much. It was too dark and sad staying in my body. There was no freedom. I had to get out.

Denial is one path that may be helpful. Just don't get lost there. Years ago I read a story about Mary Tyler Moore, a TV star known for her upbeat attitude, who was a major inspiration for her generation. Mary developed type 1 as an adult. After years with diabetes she went to a specialist with her husband, an MD. I'll use quotes but I don't have the original source. This is the conversation I remember.

"How are you?" the specialist asked.

"Oh, I'm fine," Mary chirped.

"My God, Mary," her husband broke in. "Tell him about the pain in your feet and legs. Tell him you can't sleep!" Fortunately, her informed loved one reeled her in and told her specialist what she needed.

Mary employed denial. There's also fight, flight or freeze and combinations of all three. As a child I froze, hoping to disappear. As a teen I fought, responding with "Tell me don't and I surely will." As an adult I have alternated between fight and flight.

Some of us use adversity to catapult us forward and upward. We build strength and perseverance, and take difficult but necessary steps. Doing all that you have to do to live long and well with type 1 diabetes can add meaning to your life. Having a reason to find your own truths is one of the ways diabetes may be an ally.

Real health calls for self-awareness as well as willingness to take on a challenge. You will find your own path. And as you learn, you will adjust and find better ways to be a human being with type 1 diabetes. My only warning is to stay in tune with what your body needs. Don't let high blood sugar reign.

Living with the darker aspects of diabetes is one reason many consider us warriors. Not wanting to live at war, I prefer to think of myself as a partner in a tango. *Merriam-Webster Dictionary* defines a tango as: a difficult dance in two-four time characterized by graceful posturing, frequent pointing positions, and a great variety of steps....

My life with diabetes is a difficult dance. I am often posturing, though not necessarily gracefully. There are certainly a great variety of steps I must take with my diabetes partner. But I am getting better at it.

Dancing with type 1 diabetes demands commitment, determination and the ability to adjust. Mostly we don't center our sense of self around our physical dramas. We don't think about death every day, but we might develop a deeper sense of meaning when living in its shadow. The type 1s I know or have met over time are curious and innovative people.

Completing my internship to become a Medtronic insulin pump trainer, I met a seven-year-old boy who got type 1 as an infant and was being hooked up to his first insulin pump. David had studied the pump and all its functions, inserted the different infusion sets to find the one he liked, and badgered his whole family to learn with him. He grabbed my arm and pulled me down to his height. Beaming, David confided, "My mom says as soon as they find a cure for diabetes I can take the pump apart!" Yea mom!

As we ate pizza to celebrate her son's technological advancement, David's mother patted my back and whispered, "I know you've had diabetes a long time. How are your kidneys?"

Most of our parents, spouses, siblings and close friends know how serious type 1 is and how it can impact us over time. They have probably seen that the action of injected insulin can be unpredictable, and helped you deal with highs and lows. Keep educating your personal team members. They need to know how hypoglycemia can manifest and how to assist you. They need to know how to help you, lovingly and without judgment, make choices that keep you in a healthy blood sugar range over time. When your entire circle of loved ones assists you, disaster may be forestalled.

At certain times we are close to death. Hypoglycemia can kill. So can hyperglycemia. Hypo strikes quickly and hyper most often creeps in over time.

Hypoglycemia Risk

Attempting to stay alive, many type 1s, especially people who are single, fear falling asleep because hypoglycemia might take them in the night. Parents worry about hypo in their sleeping children and set up alarm systems to alert them when their child's blood sugar falls too low. I crawled into bed for many years with blood sugar at 150, hoping that would keep me from going below 70 in the night and never waking up. Now I wear a continuous glucose monitor and an insulin pump. Both screech at me when my blood sugar gets low, and the pump shuts off insulin until I recover.

For best protection, the American Diabetes Association recommends people with diabetes keep their *average* blood sugar below 153 mg/dL—an A1c of 7%. The American Association of Clinical

Endocrinologists wants our average blood sugar even lower—at an A1c of 6½%. Many type 1s have been in jeopardy for years attempting to maintain a lower average without recurring incidents of hypoglycemia. Preventing hypoglycemia is the reason that the recommended average blood sugars for children and elders are higher than for most adults.

New technology protects us, but not completely. It sometimes fails, so low blood sugar can still overcome us even when we are plugged into technology. Hypoglycemia is one of the issues that good doctors address at every appointment.

Hyperglycemia Risk

Type 1s are also threatened with the results of high blood sugar. High blood sugar usually advances slowly into complications, but it may strike suddenly with diabetic ketoacidosis. Untreated DKA results in coma and can be fatal.

I was approaching DKA prior to my diagnosis and have come close several more times. But I didn't get all the way into coma until many years later. The first and second time I experienced DKA leading to coma I was working with herbs and other natural remedies, attempting to get off insulin. Although stopping insulin was not particularly my ambition, I lived with a healer who thought that could be done. I am grateful to have survived two episodes of DKA-induced coma.

A Cure?

Is there a cure? Several concepts occur to me that may be helpful if you contemplate curing your type 1.

First, the people proposing such an accomplishment, particularly through lifestyle changes, probably don't understand the difference between type 1 and type 2 diabetes.

Second, I believe in miracles. People report that they have cured or can cure T1D. I believe that is possible though unlikely and rare. But faith or spiritual enlightenment may result in cures.

Third, a cure may not mean healing a physical condition. A cure may be mental or emotional, but not change our need for injected insulin. In that way we may certainly be cured.

Whenever a physical cure for type 1 diabetes does arrive, let's be ready to receive it—healthy, self-aware and willing to stay in touch with our wonderful resilient bodies.

Meanwhile, with help from friends, professionals and from your own knowledge and persistence, you have survived. You have grown in awareness of how your body works. You have mastered many of the intricacies of this tango with type 1. Keep going, there will be more to learn until you leave this life—cured or not.

PART 6

WILL YOU TANGO WITH DIABETES?

CHAPTER 20

Dancing in the Dark

I always like to look on the optimistic side of life, but I am realistic enough to know that life is a complex matter.

Walt Disney
Entrepreneur, Animator, Writer, Actor and Film Producer

Optimism sustains me but I am not stupid. There's no denying that living with type 1 diabetes is hard.

I wake at 3:30 a.m. My blood sugar is at 190. I take insulin to bring it down. I cannot sleep, remembering a brief love affair in my thirties with a man who drove his motorcycle into the back of a semi. He was drunk and speeding home after the bar closed—smashed his face and lost his sight. That terrible accident happened before I met him. And when I met him I thought I already knew him—that our relationship was one of those that recur across eternity. We intertwined for a few weeks and then he moved away. Perhaps he came in this morning to help me describe what cannot be seen.

Leaving bed in spite of the hour, I pull up a friend's email that introduces the shadow side of the tango with diabetes.

"Today is my 40 year Diaversary" he wrote. "You are the only one I can tell that understands and appreciates what that means."

I regret that I am the only one he can tell. But I do understand and appreciate what it means that my friend is alive and well and employed and sane after 40 years with T1D. On my Diaversary, which is just before Halloween, I must remember to understand and appreciate myself! I too am alive and well and employed and sane.

The demands of T1D are unremitting. Every moment of every day I must remain in synch with my intricate dance partner—diabetes. While my blood sugar wanders from good to bad and back again, I tune in, make adjustments, plan ahead, meet emergencies and dance like no one is watching. No one is watching. I am on my own with this partner.

Ordinarily I dip and sway as if all is well. But when my diabetes dance becomes too much to bear—usually when my blood sugar is high—I can act the diva. If I'm alone I throw a tantrum. I stomp and kick things, scare cats and shout curses. I slam doors and scatter piles of paper. I stack insulin, demanding that my pump give me more. Then of course I plummet into hypoglycemia—which makes me paranoid and self-critical.

Some days I don't spin out of that cycle. Important projects are abandoned and I feel too wretched to take action. On those days I hate having diabetes.

Trying to soothe myself I recall examples of other people's fiascos with T1D. A diabetes educator I will call Jane described dancing with friends at a party and going outside for fresh air. She lost awareness for a moment and found herself lying on the ground. When she was discovered, Jane called for her boyfriend—who knew she needed to drink juice and bring her blood sugar up. Jane had had diabetes for many years and worked with it professionally. But dancing and laughing, perhaps drinking alcohol without food, brought her blood sugar dangerously low. It can happen to any of us at any time. Training our loved ones helps. If her boyfriend hadn't known what to do, another partygoer could have called 911 and caused unnecessary turmoil for Jane.

Another T1D proved her mettle on a Mexican dive trip. Laura made sure her blood sugar was high before every dive so she wouldn't get hypoglycemic underwater. That was a wise choice, although of course the experts say we aren't supposed to do such a thing. Keep that damned sugar inside the lines at all times they insist. But their rules don't always work. Type 1 is inconstant. We have to think for ourselves and find our own ways. We learn and we adapt. That's how we benefit and advance.

Yes, we do have technological help and it is a benefit. Some of us have setups called closed loop systems that mimic the pancreas— stopping insulin when we're low and adding insulin when we're high. However, we still have to intervene, and nothing manmade works as well as a healthy human body. Scientists, especially those with T1D family members, are trying to create miraculous inventions to end T1D. For now, our technology remains limited.

Those who don't have T1D don't always understand how

imperfect our machines are, or that they are just machines. A young medical intern joined the staff in the clinic where I was working, saw my pump and burbled, "Isn't that wonderful! Don't you love your pump?" I wasn't as kind as I like to be. I hit her with, "I don't love my pump. Do you love your computer, your cell phone, your stethoscope?"

My pump is a tool for which I am grateful. It serves me well but it also reminds me of a needy pet. Pump wearers have infusion sets taped to our bodies that hold in place a cannula inserted under the skin. The pump connects to the infusion set with an 18", 23", 32" or 43" plastic tube that delivers insulin. Tubing catches on doorknobs and desk corners and my cats love to bite it! And say goodbye to sleeping in the nude or a lightweight nightgown while wearing a pump. The demanding little thing is heavy and needs to clamp onto a solid piece of clothing.

Avoiding that connection is a reason many T1Ds wear a tubeless Omnipod. Both pump infusion sets and Omnipods need to be changed every two to three days. CGM sensors are also inserted under the skin but last 10-14 days before being peeled off and replaced.

Unlike phones or computers, diabetes technology is attached to us and has to be worn every day. We have to avoid breaking it, remember to charge it, keep it clean and dry, and find a way to pay for expensive supplies and updates. Our pumps and CGMs scream at us when our blood sugar goes off course, or when we have to change infusion sets. Tech support insists I can't turn off my Tandem pump's piercing alarms when it's out of insulin, so I bury it under my mattress when I want to postpone the steps to set it all up again.

"I know! I know!" I shout as it screeches, hastening out of

earshot. Once it's muffled I inject insulin with a syringe and live pump-free for a few hours.

When I go to hot springs or a beach, I have to figure out how long I can be unhooked without needing insulin. Then I have to figure out how to safely stash my pump and CGM monitor where they won't be stepped on or knocked into the water or sand, where they won't overheat or be stolen.

Any activity, making love for example, is complicated by these attachments. Where do you put the damned pump so it will neither interfere nor go flying? I can disconnect from the pump and put it under the pillow, but the infusion set on my abdomen still intrudes.

Finding the best place to attach my pump causes ongoing upset. Pumps are both heavy and destructible, and not all pump clips are foolproof. My wardrobe has significantly changed and still my pump detaches and whacks me or pulls out my infusion set, or the screen cracks when it hits the floor. For the most part I wear jeans with an over-shirt and pajamas with pockets. My denim jeans and flannel PJs have stable waistbands to secure my pump. And a shirt that's spacious and not tucked in lets me hide my pump and wear my CGM unrestricted.

With my wardrobe and technology secured, I can consider going out!

For civilized outings, like a celebratory dinner, I arrive only after having investigated the menu online, spoken with the chef by phone and worked hard to balance my blood sugar so I can eat what I want without spiking. Often I get hypoglycemic about the time I need to leave the house. That means I have to eat or drink something sweet to bring my blood sugar up to normal, and spoil my appetite.

Once I was treated by a generous friend to a lovely lunch at a famous restaurant. Chatting happily, I ordered my meal and reached for my insulin pump. No pump! In my hurry to shower and dress and rush to meet my friend, I forgot to clip my pump back on. And I brought a fancy small purse that didn't have my emergency kit in it—no insulin and no syringe. I considered staying put and letting my blood sugar go up without insulin but couldn't relax with that plan. I left my friend sipping her wine while I rushed home to grab my pump.

Mistakes are often more than irritating. They can be costly and even deadly. Costly and deadly mistakes are addressed elsewhere. But irritating mistakes are part of life. I apply my mental repair techniques, and stay on a positive track—not always successfully.

Most days following the steps that keep me alive and well is simply what I do, like brushing my teeth and combing my hair. I don't acknowledge the demands of my diabetes self-care. I just do what's necessary. Other days I hate diabetes. I hate what I have to do. I hate my life. And that may translate into hating myself.

This forever dilemma has shaped me. While most of us put on a public face that hides our challenges and fears, T1Ds must reach deeper. Our condition is essentially invisible. Yet even a few hours without paying attention to it has consequences. I occasionally feel like nothing is in my control. Even when I do everything right my blood sugar may still take me into a harmful range. And my friends, coworkers or loved ones may see me disintegrate and wonder why I am always late, or why I am short-tempered. It helps to let them know when I'm in a *can't-win* mood with my diabetes.

How do your family and friends respond when you are struggling to manage your invisible condition? Do they even know that diabetes is the reason you aren't ready or burst into a tantrum?

Moments of struggle might be alleviated simply by reducing the need to be perfect. Although I am almost always 15 minutes late, I am getting better about stopping, taking long breaths, smiling and loving myself while addressing my diabetes needs. All I have to do is take insulin, check my blood sugar, drink juice, or change my CGM. That's not so hard. I can slow down and do it.

Communication is harder, but I can manage that too. I may turn to my beloved and say, "I need a few minutes to deal with diabetes stuff." Or I can be my beloved and say that to myself. Diabetes becomes my ally again when I slow down and attend to my precious human body.

Sometimes I envy those who don't have to pay such close attention. Most of the time it doesn't even occur to me. I rely on my knowledge and my versatile body. My days as a mountaineer beautifully trained me to be prepared. I am not a person with diabetes who has to fend off disaster. I am a wise veteran walking through life with helpful awareness.

Coming back to my small-city home after a wilderness trek many years ago, I ambled through the neighborhood with a friend. A large scary dog came leaping and barking at us and my friend jumped into the street. I continued on the sidewalk.

"You didn't even react!" he shouted at me.

"The dog was behind a fence," I shrugged.

Staying sane and calm with all that's going on is a never-ending enterprise. But it makes me a good human. And remaining angry at my condition, my body or myself puts me in a terrible mood and leaves me feeling hopeless and victimized. What's the way out?

Beliefs count. In my adult life I have circled around diverse spiritual and physical philosophies to find what serves me. I never had an exciting or dramatic spiritual awakening but I clearly remember standing on the sidewalk in front of my apartment in Boulder, Colorado as I approached age 30. In my hands was the book *Yoga, Youth & Reincarnation* by Jess Stearn. That book introduced me to the idea that my soul advanced through lifetimes. Standing there, I decided that I would believe in reincarnation, because it gave me perspective. It gave me hope and consolation. It provided meaning for tough times I had experienced. Whatever had happened to me, including type 1 diabetes, I decided, was for my highest good. It might even be true that I chose it as a source of enlightenment.

The thought of gratitude sneaks in—another philosophy that I have adopted. Staying in gratitude and knowing that diabetes aids in my spiritual development as well as my physical wellbeing, I am better able to face its challenges.

My philosophies create a path I can follow through dark and light. Diabetes can feel like a total eclipse of the sun. Many of the inspirational quotes I've collected over the years have to do with staying in the light. But some days it's hard to find the light.

On a good day, especially when out walking, I am grateful that I am mobile and without pain. My eyes have been extensively worked on, but I can see. I can read and write and drive to work. In many ways I am blessed.

I am not perfect and not always in tune with higher awareness. I am disorderly, impatient and I curse a lot. My home is untidy. A former friend told me my car looked like a dump truck. But I don't indulge in sweets. I don't overeat. I restrict carbs. I exercise. I meet regularly with an MD, an endocrinologist, an ophthalmologist, a diabetes educator, a naturopath and a bodyworker. I take vitamins and minerals. I attend seminars on self-improvement. My average blood sugar is in the recommended range.

Still the path is devious. I rarely speak about my diabetes to people without it. Like my friend said about his Diaversary, who would understand? But I talk to myself about it.

People with diabetes are everyday wizards, each with their own magic. At work I tell my diabetes clients to find their own way and count on themselves. Those who make it two years or 10 years or 40 years, are resilient, determined, both imperfect and strong in very individual ways. We don't get to fight a disease like cancer and recover or die. We manage diabetes every day for the rest of our lives or die. How? Why? That's for you to determine. But you can do it and it's worth it and it helps if diabetes is your partner rather than your adversary. Although everything changes and we must adapt, we have a central unwavering self and a destiny that guides us.

There is always more to do and more to discover and more to comprehend. My CGM beeps. I have been writing for a couple hours, no food or drink, but my blood sugar is 232. I take insulin. For another hour I edit my words and prep for a meeting with my mentor. Still no food, only coffee. BG 330. Coffee and stress—more aspects of blood sugar control to consider. No blame. Just life with T1D.

Let nothing come between you and the light.

Henry David Thoreau
Naturalist, Essayist, Poet, and Philosopher

CHAPTER 21

Where's Your Joy?

People are always blaming their circumstances for what they are. I don't believe in circumstances. The people who get on in this world are the people who get up and look for the circumstances they want and if they can't find them, make them.

George Bernard Shaw
Irish Playwright, Critic and Political Activist

I do believe in circumstances, but Shaw's quote reminds me that I create my response to what comes to me. When I get circumstances I don't want—like having type 1 diabetes—I do all I can to find what good that circumstance brings me. Turning a bad circumstance into a beneficial one is how I have framed my T1D for more than 60 years. Perhaps you are considering that stance as you finish this book.

Recently I acknowledged that type 1 diabetes has brought me a rich life. Now I want to make my life even richer, so the circumstance I must make for myself is to experience more joy.

Having a more joyful life has been important to me for quite a while but I haven't known what to do about it. I used to think joy had to be a big thing—that I had to stand in a beam of light falling from heaven, filled with love and appreciation without a hint of pain or sorrow. Not having experienced that in my life, I thought I was lacking joy. Frustrated with that thought, I got curious and looked at my life more closely. I noticed a softer, more subtle kind of joy.

Joy fills me on a quiet morning at home hearing the baby birds in their nest in my mulberry tree screeching to be fed. Joy is the warmth of my tuxedo cat curled up on my toes while I'm writing. Joy is clean bare counters when I've washed all my dishes. And joy warms my heart when I drive down La Bajada Hill on my way to work, and see my beautiful world spread out before me. I love living where the mountains rise protectively at my back and the plains and the sky extend forever.

I'm learning to understand and embrace what joy is for me, which is proving to be as important as managing my blood sugar! My ambition is to accept whatever emotions and difficulties arise while loving myself, my life, and my crazy diabetes body. Not easy, but what an excellent doorway to greater joy.

- Where does your joy show up?

- Is it enough?

- Do you want to make joy more of a priority?

Because T1D can be so much to manage, joy can get pushed to the edges of your life. That is understandable but it doesn't have to be that way. Consider what your partnership with diabetes has brought you. Has it even occurred to you that type 1 diabetes might be your greatest inspiration? Maybe diabetes has led you through hard times to accomplishment, confidence and contentment.

Assuming that you have settled into good control, or are working to get there, you are making healthy choices. You eat conscientiously. You keep moving. You handle upsets. You have a great team. Your diabetes gear works and you have backup. Any complications you have are well controlled and you have made peace with the changes they have caused. Perhaps you are already living a life you consider joyful.

Perhaps you aren't there yet. Whether your diabetes self-care is solid or not, you may want greater satisfaction. Type 1 has pushed you to develop self-discipline and create a healthy well-balanced life. Observers may even consider you courageous. But you might not feel courageous, or at all joyful. What else does your destiny call you to fulfill?

I know that I have not expressed all that's in me. Important messages are still making their way into my active brain. Gaining pride in myself and knowing there's more has upped my joy.

On my monumental 60th birthday I knew that I was missing something in my life. I decided I wanted to spend more time in nature—particularly sleeping on the ground under the stars, and I wanted to be writing for publication. I admitted that I had let those essential experiences go, and brought writing and camping back into my life.

I joined Great Old Broads for Wilderness, a national grassroots organization that works to preserve and protect wild lands. I gratefully convened with the Broads for campouts with a purpose. Being in wild places soothes and liberates me. I feel more myself in a quiet stand of trees than anywhere else. I love waking at daylight enclosed in my sleeping bag and waiting for warm sunlight to make its way to my side of the valley. Even as a child, I felt lovingly surrounded and uplifted by evergreen branches overhead and the scent of crushed pine needles beneath my feet. At home I stand in the dirt, put a hand on my mulberry tree and take a few breaths before driving to work.

Making writing a priority again, I published articles in a national dietitian's magazine on celiac disease and traveling with type 1 diabetes. And I wrote for a local magazine about special places nearby that I love and people can visit, including Pecos and Bandelier national monuments. Both are beautiful places for walking through the remains of ancient civilizations. Bandelier has cliff dwellings carved from volcanic tuff. And the Pecos ruins include a towering restored adobe church among buried dwellings and kivas that were part of an ancient Pueblo trading center.

Besides having my work published, the act of writing brings me joy and opens the door to greater learning and fulfillment. I compile research and my own thoughts, pulling together everything I know about a topic. Then, like a sculptor carving a statue, I chip and hack and smooth my words into a readable form. The result of my writing also adds joy, especially when a reader finds it helpful.

Moments of Joy
Besides outdoor time and writing, there is a third pathway to joy for me, one that is simpler yet still profound—living in the moment.

I may feel that kind of joy pulling on hand-knit socks, eating an avocado sandwich, walking with Dawna and her old dog Gus who loves me and I love back, or sleeping in until I am truly rested and ready to get up.

When I survey my life and think about how I experience joy, for the most part I am satisfied. I know that joy is my creation, and I no longer find it too big to achieve. I recognize my very own style of joyfulness and know it is always available. I don't even have to create an event or go on a quest. Joy can mean loving what is.

Listening to a talk as I fell asleep last night, I was reminded to live in anticipation of what's good ahead rather than fearing what might be bad. When I anticipate goodness I actually feel the difference in myself and my life. I am joyful and confident. I can, and I will, enrich each day. I slow my breath, relax my shoulders and look up from my computer. My cat Baxter squeezes onto my soft writing chair to cuddle me.

I will start my day tomorrow taking time to look out my window at the huge green leaves shading my home, capped by a turquoise sky, while enjoying a perfect creamy cup of coffee.

The potential for joy is in me and in you and in each one of us. Our thoughts, our feelings and our beliefs belong to us. We create our lives. We live in our own circles of awareness. Joy is occasionally a huge gift—like a new baby or falling in love. But often joy is a grand moment in an ordinary day.

How can a person with a demanding, expensive, 24/7, life-threatening condition like type 1 diabetes be joyful? That, like every other aspect of being a human, is up to you.

Top 10 Life List

Joy may not be part of your thinking right now. Or it might be a hope you have without believing you can find it. Like me on a certain birthday, you might one day discover that your life is incomplete. A review of your values might be helpful.

- Are you living the way you want to live?

- What is joyful in your life right now?

- How might you acknowledge and even enhance that feeling?

- How might you shape your thoughts and your actions to create opportunities for greater joy?

Many people formulate a bucket list of things to do before they die. I prefer to think of a life list that includes my essential values. Having that list in my mind, or even written down, reminds me what's important. And it may push me to change my ways from time to time.

My sister Nancy surrounds herself with beauty. Her home is lovely and so is her yard. She watches birds bathing in a fountain outside the window as she checks her email. She cooks and bakes for neighbors and loved ones, setting the dining table with exquisite plates and glasses and silver, folded cloth napkins and tiny individual salt and pepper shakers. Even in her denim skirt and tee shirt she wears gold and diamond bracelets, rings and necklaces.

She is a canny and thrifty shopper and riches didn't fall into her life. Nancy established priorities and took steps to create and maintain her beautiful surroundings. She and her husband moved around the country for work opportunities and took jobs or lived places they didn't always like. But they had a vision. When Nancy and I visit back and forth, we always go shopping. She likes to visit jewelry stores, where her treasures are greatly admired, and she is able to converse knowledgeably. I am happy just to be with her. On one visit she asked whether I liked jewelry. "Yes, I do," I answered, "but it's not in my top 10."

That conversation led me to consider my life list.

My top 10 values include unstructured time, being in nature, organic food, hiking, having enough money, and staying well with diabetes. Living exactly where I want to live on earth is in my top 10. So is having an SUV I can sleep in if back country weather explodes, and maintaining a strong body that lets me be mobile without pain. Spirituality is in my top 10. Learning more about myself is on my list too. My expendable earnings are applied to seminars and conferences and mentoring and coaching. Being able to apply what I learn and continue to change is on my list.

I am already past 10, but it's a helpful way to think about how I use my time and my resources. Some items on my *most important* list support my survival and others bring me joy.

Having established that joyfulness matters to me, there's the challenge of continuing. Like everyone else, listing a desired outcome in my top 10 does not mean I give it all the attention it deserves. Although spending time in nature is in my top 10, I don't get outside often enough, not even into my yard to sit under the mulberry tree and watch the sky change. My type 1 self-care is vital. Yet I may slide by without giving it my best—ignoring blood sugar checks, eating badly, etc. And when I am cranky and resistant, joy sinks through the cracks. I have to re-commit myself to both the must-dos and the want-tos. As in other places in this book, I remind myself and you that we are human and have to begin again and again to create and re-create our lives to optimize our type 1 care and our joy.

Consider your top 10 life list.

- Are you living with what's most important to you?

- If one of your values has been ignored, how might you add it to what you already know and do?

- Are there moments in your day when you appreciate and even thank yourself for what you have chosen?

- Or has your joy been so well hidden that you can't find it?

Look around. Walk through your home. Give yourself the gift of what you already have. And promise yourself to attend to whatever you have neglected. Your joy may quicken as you enliven your top 10 life list.

Making Good Out of Bad

Despite good intentions, life may get in your way. Over my diabetes educator career I have worked in communities that had a high rate of type 2 diabetes. Yet diabetes and self-care were not on peoples' top 10 lists. That greatly concerned me.

Especially during the pandemic, many of my clients were hanging on with tremendous courage but little room for anything beyond survival. They were not making enough money, had to feed their extended families, couldn't make car payments, and lived in homes that didn't always protect them from the weather. Diabetes didn't make their lists—even though many of their family members had diabetes.

However, those people often had tremendous joy in their lives. They had fulfilling religious and cultural practices. They had close-knit families. And they worried about me! When first invited to attend tribal festivities at a nearby Pueblo, I arrived at my friend Noreen's 3-bedroom ranch house too early. Grandpa was watching TV in his pajamas. Little grandchildren ran screaming through the house, and sleepy adults peeked at me from behind doors. Noreen gathered everyone up to dress and prepare for the day. I washed dishes and chopped vegetables for the feast later. When everyone was ready, we drove into the village and watched the beautiful prayerful dancing, with breaks at Noreen's mother's home on the plaza to serve feast day foods to dancers and observers.

Driving home I savored my singular life and worried that Noreen had so many people in her house and not much time for herself or to care for her diabetes. At work the next day she hugged me and revealed that she and her family were sorry that I was so alone. They didn't want me to be lonely and invited me to visit any time. My awareness was blown open by their generous and grateful hearts.

Thinking of you who are reading this, no matter how hard it is, please find a way to keep your blood sugar in a healthy range. And let simple joys help you. Diabetes may feel like the worst thing that ever happened to you. Diabetes may be a curse you ignore, you suffer from, you despise, you resist or you fight. Your life may feel impossibly difficult. Let it be easier. Find ways to love yourself, care for your diabetes and bring in joy.

Many years ago I heard a poem read on the radio. I was fussing around my house trying to organize, and when I heard that poem I sat down hard and cried. I have never found the poem again, but I remember the image it created. It was written by a woman in isolation in a Russian prison who had a tiny window high above her head. She woke to see the morning light shine through the window and followed its imprint across the walls surrounding her. Watching the light come and go through that window brought her joy. It probably saved her sanity.

Philosophers say that life is hard. Life with type 1 diabetes is certainly hard. I worry and I resist and rebel. I have days when I actually spit out, "Life sucks and then you die." But I don't do that every day, and I do believe that choosing how I respond to challenges is my primary freedom. My response to life and to diabetes is up to me.

Outer world changes flare up around us and have effects. When Covid-19 arrived, one of the spiritual leaders I listen to called Covid the ultimate pop-quiz for those of us seeking deeper awareness. With job loss, isolation, potential illness or death, and ongoing insecurity, I wondered, how will people with type 1 diabetes fare on this quiz?

- How will those of us who have lost work and are unable to bring in money not just survive but go beyond?

- What about T1Ds who are deemed essential and must work in danger, T1Ds who cannot afford to buy insulin or food, T1Ds enduring racial discrimination?

- How will we remember who we are and continue to allow joy to peek in?

Life is not simple or easy for any of us. But we have the opportunity to create appreciation and happiness no matter how we live, no matter what life throws at us. Your way to create the life you want is different from anyone else's. As in the quote I started with, "The people who get on in this world are the people who get up and look for the circumstances they want and if they can't find them, make them."

Appreciate your diabetes. Step into that tango. Make your life circumstances both healthy and joyful. Why not?

The End

Now you know how I address my capricious and powerful friend T1D. And you have examples of people with T1D who are living adventurous lives. Perhaps one of my stories has inspired you to consider your diabetes differently.

If you are embracing new behaviors, I have been told again and again—take small steps.

Here's a life example. My friend Ava is an organizer. She helped me address my overwhelm about spring housecleaning by describing in detail a book she had both listened to and read. She advised me to read the book and to use the templates the author provided to organize my life and make plans.

I could not face that! I hated the idea of reading that book, filling out forms or making plans. But Ava simplified what she had learned, advising me to break my huge housecleaning challenge into doable bits and time them.

"Pick one small part of your plan," she said, "Set a realistic time limit, and do it."

Inspired by our conversation I started with 10 minutes hanging up all the jackets and fleece vests piled in my living room. Doing that was so satisfying that I decided to wash clothes. I did not set a time frame and I did not stick to one small task. Once started I kept going and washed three loads of clothes! After sorting, washing, drying, folding and putting away three washer loads of clothes, I lost momentum for the whole next day.

Knowing that I am always tempted to do too much, I need to remind myself, "Start small. Stay small." How might I adapt that approach for health steps?

Because I am so content curled up with cats and laptop computer at home, I struggle to walk regularly. I have to set pleasant goals for walking the recommended 30 minutes a day five days a week. If I drive downtown to check my PO Box, I circle Federal Place three times on foot appreciating the giant trees, which adds up to a pleasant 30 minutes. If I want to buy a lottery ticket a mile away hoping to win $100,000 to remodel my home, I will get out and walk.

Setting a timer and keeping my goals realistic helps. T1D encourages me, demanding that I attend to my wonderful and needy body. To maintain comprehensive self-care, instead of arguing with myself or resisting, I separate my tasks into chunks I can handle. Knowing I need extra time, I may get up earlier or shorten my to-do list so I can complete my health chores and take a walk.

If you are not yet where you want to be with your self-care, how might you shift your approach or adopt new health behaviors? You are in charge. And choosing to stay well with T1D is holistic, providing opportunities to enrich your life and find greater meaning.

Take action deliberately. Know that you can do this. It is worth it. You don't need to be perfect. Whatever you do will make a difference. Your health care must-dos may lead you to organize and simplify more effectively than you otherwise would. And you will find your own way! With good medical advice and support from within, you can live a full and adventurous life as you are, with T1D. You can dance beautifully with one of life's most demanding partners.

Keep learning. Stay curious. Have a plan and start over every single morning. Tango with diabetes.

The great thing about life is you always have to start over. No matter how many meals you've eaten, nights you've slept, breaths you've taken, you always have to start over.

Marty Rubin
Gay Activist, Journalist and Author

I hope my book has encouraged you to find your own ways to create better health and happiness with your diabetes. Please visit KarenMeadowsDiabetes.com for more resources and events.

Printed in the USA
CPSIA information can be obtained
at www.ICGtesting.com
JSHW081105241023
50721JS00004B/94